SHIFU SAID
Tai Chi, Qigong, and the Chinese Health Culture

Janice Doppler

DEDICATION

This book is dedicated to WEI WEN TAO and JEAN CHU without whom Shifu could not have accomplished what she did.

CONTENTS

INTRODUCTION

Master Lijun Cheng dreamed of writing a series of books for Americans - tai chi, qigong, Chinese health culture, and an autobiography. Multiple students reached for that dream with her. I was the last who tried. Our work was fueled by a shared determination to preserve ancient Chinese wisdom. Shifu's job was passing wisdom accumulated through decades of study and practice. Mine was reshaping it into an English format for westerners. Together, we aimed to build a bridge from past to present.

Language differences made the work quite difficult. Frequent use of translation devices was necessary when we worked alone. Sometimes Yaping Sun, Shuk Chan, Wen Tao Wei, and most frequently Jean Chu translated for us. Many times we thought we'd agreed on something only to find out we'd totally misunderstood each other. We were both exhausted by the end of each work session.

The pace of our work was inconsistent. Periods of weekly day-long work sessions were punctuated by months without working together. During the down times, I organized my notes from post-qigong question and answer periods into content crafted to reveal Shifu's teachings. It was tough going since details about how to do qigong were randomly interspersed with teachings about lifestyle practices and other topics.

Other than the story of her life, which was published in *Healing Bodies, Healing Hearts with Tai Chi Chuan and Qigong*, we never got close to accomplishing the task that we considered to be our shared mission. After Shifu's sudden death in 2014, I wondered whether our work was waste of time because all we did was pile building material on the bank of the river and never started the bridge. Did years of work mean anything? The challenges and joys of our collaboration and my personal daily qigong practice and study of Chinese philosophy that Shifu inspired made me a different person than who I was before it all started. Was the bridge we built just a bridge from who I was to who I am? Could that possibly be enough? It is time to admit that it is not enough. It is time to share the material Shifu and I piled on the bank of the river.

This book is aimed at a small audience - former students at the International Center for Harmony and Living Arts founded by Master Lijun Cheng. Content comes from varied sources - narrative woven class notes from random instruction, lecture notes, and some from notes written at home after class. I stayed as close as possible to the words Shifu actually spoke in hopes that her voice will shine through the words on the page.

My hope is that each reader of this book can find material to reinforce bridges already under construction in the lives of each of Shifu's students.

1 YANG LUCHAN TO CHENG LIJUN

Shifu Cheng rarely spoke of the Yang style tai chi chuan lineage; however, she gave Center for Harmony students the following account. "According to legend, tai chi chuan was originated by Daoist Zhang San Feng (*Chang San Feng*) who studied at Shaolin Temple for a few years before going to Wudan Mountain. Zhang San Feng's disciple, Wang Zongyue, renamed "long boxing" as tai chi chuan and taught it to Chen Wangting (1580-1660 C.E.) who founded Chen style tai chi chuan. Many generations later, Yang Luchan (1799-1872 C.E.) secretly observed the tai chi practice of Chen family members for whom he worked in Chen Village, Henan Province. After being caught watching he demonstrated what he had learned on his own and Chen Changxing (*Ch'en Chang-hsing*) (1771-1853 C.E.) formally accepted Yang Luchan as his student. After completing his studies with Chen Changxing, Yang Luchan modified the Chen style by making it slower and more graceful. This marked the founding of Yang Style Tai Chi. Yang Luchan became the best martial artist in China and was invited to Beijing to teach the emperor and officials of the Qing Dynasty. Yang Luchan taught his sons Banhou (*Pan-hou*) and Jianhou (*Chien-hou*). Yang Jianhou taught his son, Yang Cheng Fu (1883-1936,) who became the third-generation lineage holder. Yang Cheng Fu, appointed multiple fourth-generation lineage holders including Cui Yishi who taught Liu Gao Ming who Cui named as one of several fifth-generation lineage holders. Liu Gao Ming appointed me as one among multiple sixth-generation lineage holders."

In 1979, Liu Gao Ming was assigned as Head Coach at the Beijing Consulate, where he taught many prominent people including Barbara Bush the Twenty-Four Form during her husband's tenure as United States Ambassador to China. Liu Gao Ming told a story about Barbara Bush in an interview published in China's *Soul of Martial Arts Magazine* in February 2001. "At the beginning, I followed my superior's instruction to speak little and practice much in class then leave as soon as class is over. Later, I noticed a tall, middle-aged woman who was very eager to learn and who practiced very seriously. After one round of practice, she was in a sweat. She continued practicing even when class was over. If she was unsure about anything during practice, she asked questions through an interpreter – the wife of the Austrian ambassador to China. Through the interpreter, I knew that the hard-working student was Barbara, wife of Ambassador George H. W. Bush. By the time of the class graduation she could practice the Twenty-Four Form very well. Generally speaking, the Snake Creeps Down form is a difficult move especially for middle-aged people with no experience, but Mrs. Bush could do this form very well with her lower body firm and leg fully stretched while keeping her upper body straight. For the performance at the class graduation ceremony, only two students were elected to represent each continent because the stage was small. Mrs. Bush was elected as one of the North American representatives. Mrs. Bush had not realized this event would include playing tai chi so she did not bring her tai chi shoes; however, she was so excited to be selected that she took off her high-heeled shoes and got on the stage. That brought a great cheer from the audience and laughter from Mr. Bush."

Shifu was reluctant to discuss her personal experience with learning tai chi chuan. Initially, she said "I took classes twice a week. I practiced in the park every morning. I helped other people learn. With tai chi chuan, the only thing is practicing. The more you practice the more you learn. Other than that, there is not much to talk about." After being pushed for more information, Shifu Cheng shared the following story of how she learned tai chi and eventually became the sixth-generation lineage holder of Yang style tai chi:

My parents arranged for me to attend a martial arts school to learn Shaolin Fist (*hongquan*) when I was seven years old. I had an aptitude for martial arts and quickly became one of the top students in spite of being the smallest. I combined my martial arts skills with what my mother taught me about ensuring justice and developed a reputation for protecting children who were being bullied. Any time bullying began, someone would run for me. I'd verbally challenge bullies to stop being hurtful and if they refused, I used martial arts to force them to stop. After a while, older boys ran away as soon as they saw me coming to assist a child being bullied.

In the early 1960s when I was in my mid-twenties, I was assigned a job teaching the government-mandated exercise routine performed by every worker each morning. As part of my responsibilities, I was expected to know as much about physical activity as possible so I began learning tai chi chuan. First, I learned the Standard Chinese National Tai Chi Chuan Twenty-Four Form developed in 1956 by tai chi chuan masters Chu Guiting, Cai Longyun, Fu Zhongwen, and Zhang Yu who were commissioned by the government's National Physical Culture and Sports Commission to create a simple tai chi chuan form that could be practiced by the general public. Later, I learned other forms. Students were required to pass a test before being permitted to learn a new form. The test was much like the way I test students at Center for Harmony with the student being tested performing alone while classmates watch. Small mistakes that were corrected did not mean failure. I shook inside when I was tested.

I attended two three-hour tai chi chuan classes each week at the Workers' Cultural Palace (*Wenhua Gong*) located between Tiananmen Square and what is now known as the Forbidden City. It was originally a temple where the emperors of the Ming and Qing dynasties worshipped. It included a beautiful garden with enormous trees that were over a thousand years old. People gathered there each morning to practice tai chi chuan, tai chi sword, or other activities. Chinese opera singers practiced there too each morning! It was a calm, peaceful place and I practiced there any time the opportunity arose. I miss that part of Beijing more than any other place.

I longed to learn from Liu Gao Ming who was one among many teachers at the Cultural Palace. He was famous throughout China since he had won many national martial arts competitions and was a fifth-generation lineage holder of Yang style tai chi chuan. He had students in many countries and taught only a few advanced groups at the Workers' Cultural Palace. When our paths occasionally crossed, we chatted informally.

My learning tai chi chuan was interrupted when the Cultural Revolution swept through China. I was branded as an anti-revolutionary class enemy and was sentenced to heavy labor in the countryside. Two years later the political climate improved enough so that I could return to Beijing; however, I was still labeled a class enemy and was vulnerable to beatings at any time. I secretly practiced tai chi chuan and qigong in my home. I was assigned a low status job that was intended to humiliate and isolate me, but I consider myself lucky because it enabled me to resume tai chi and qigong classes at the Worker's Cultural Palace.

One day during the 1970s, while practicing tai chi I experienced so much pain in my back that I could barely stand up. I went to the hospital and was diagnosed with mediastinal cancer, a tumor between my lung and heart, with a prognosis of death within six months. I refused to accept the prognosis and undertook an intense healing regime. I arose at 5:30 each morning for an hour of tai chi and an hour of a standing qigong called *zhan zhuang* to which I added a healing breathing technique normally used during sitting qigong. I created a simple tai chi Twelve Form because I did not have the strength to do the kicks in the traditional long form. When I played tai chi, pressure from the tumor felt like a knife in my back with each inhalation. Even though I rarely got to bed before 1:00 am, each day ended with an hour of sitting qigong. During these sessions it often felt like ice melting inside me. When I returned to the physician six months after the diagnosis, the tumor had shrunk to half its previous size. Now, more than thirty years later, there is no sign of the tumor. I use my Twelve Form to teach beginners.

Liu Gao Ming was impressed that I continued attending classes in spite of having cancer and my long-time wish of being accepted as his student came true. By 1978, society had become more open and he had enough political power to risk coming to my home in spite of my label as an anti-revolutionary class enemy. He taught me privately on Sundays in addition to the twice weekly classes at the Worker's Palace. He eventually initiated me as his disciple.

On the day I immigrated to the United States in 1994, Liu Gao Ming drove me to the airport. He encouraged me to teach in America and gave me ten plastic collapsible swords that I currently use when I teach sword. At that point, I did not intend to teach; however, after arriving in the United States I quickly noticed that many people wanted to learn tai chi, but many teachers did not truly understand it. I was invited to a party where they did tai chi chuan, but it was not really tai chi chuan. I saw that some people were learning only from videotapes and I worried that they would not understand enough to reap the health benefits of tai chi chuan and might even damage their bodies. A Chinese man who claimed to have extensive background in tai chi chuan invited me to teach at his school, but his skills were poor and he admitted to me that none of his claims of expertise were true. I was upset by what I saw so I wanted to begin teaching tai chi chuan in addition to the qigong I had already begun teaching.

I traveled to China obtain formal permission from Liu Gao Ming to teach in the United States. He appointed me as a Sixth Generation Yang Style Lineage holder at that point. I returned to the United States where I taught at an ever-expanding list of senior centers, churches, and fitness centers in Connecticut and Massachusetts. In 1999, at the age of sixty-one, I established the International Center for Harmony and Living Arts in western Massachusetts.

2 TAI CHI CHUAN OR TAI CHI?

Tai chi chuan (*taijiquan*) is the name of the martial art which, according to legend, was developed by Daoist master Zhang San Feng (*Chang San Feng*). *Chuan* means fist so tai chi chuan means tai chi fist. People often call the martial art tai chi, but tai chi in English (*taiji* in pin yin) is actually a philosophical term that has deep meaning in Chinese cosmology. Tai chi (*taiji*) is made of two Chinese words. Tai can mean big (*da*) if written 大 and small (*tai*) if written 太. Ji (*ji*) means to the ultimate or to the extreme whether the direction of movement is toward its ultimate largeness or ultimate smallness. Tai chi chuan is more than a martial art since it incorporates philosophy and culture. Understanding the underlying philosophy and culture contributes to learning the martial art.

Tai Chi Chuan – A Martial Art

Tai chi chuan is a martial art that combines the hardness of steel with softness of cotton and emphasizes use of intention rather than force or strength. Turning the waist, the axis of all tai chi chuan movement, can generate a great deal of force. According to tai chi classic texts, "four ounces controls a thousand pounds."

Tai chi chuan is a healing exercise that promotes circulation within the body via constant internal and external circling movements which correspond to the cyclical movements within the universe. Turning the waist promotes circulation within meridians. Keeping the tailbone tucked when performing tai chi chuan forms improves the flow of energy in meridians between the bottom of the spine (*hui yin*) and crown of the head (*bai hui*).

Tai chi chuan's slow, beautiful movements coordinated with rhythmic breathing yield internal benefits that other sports lack. Since tai chi chuan consumes less yang energy than other types of aerobic exercise it preserves the original energy (*yuan qi*) with which a person is born. Performing tai chi chuan strengthens the legs which is important since legs are often the first thing to weaken as a person ages. Tai chi chuan promotes calmness and relaxation which, in turn, improves one's personality.

Tai chi chuan developed as a martial art because people had to fight with their hands since guns were not available. Modern people fight with guns and don't need to fight with their hands. Modern people need health. Although playing tai chi chuan alone has health benefits, it is most effective at promoting healing and preventing disease part of a package that combines a philosophy of life grounded in cultivating virtue, qigong, and following the Chinese health culture in which eating, drinking, emotions, exercise, sleeping, sexual activity, and clothing choices are aligned with the rhythms of nature.

Tai chi chuan is not a regular sport because its circular movements stimulate tai chi organs and generates tai chi energy. Its movements balance yin and yang and the five elements or five energetic phases which are important concepts in traditional Chinese medicine. It incorporates the eight trigrams (*bagua*) described in the following section.

Tai Chi – Philosophy and Cosmology

Many Americans are familiar with the tai chi symbol (*taijitu*) and have heard of the *Book of Changes*, often known by its Chinese name *Yi Jing* (*I Ching*), but few know the philosophy behind these concepts. The tai chi symbol was developed during the Han Dynasty *(206 B.C.E – 220 C.E.)* to represent varied aspects of Chinese cosmology. The motion of the universe is depicted in the yin-yang symbol. The entire symbol represents the Dao. The dark areas represent yin and light areas represent yang. The principles illustrated in this symbol apply to the dynamics of yin and yang that impact everything in the universe. Heaven and earth comprise the large universe. The human body is a small universe that parallels the dynamics of the large universe. The symbol represents yin and yang remaining balanced during constant motion requires constant adjustment between increase and decrease of yin and yang. The symbol is a two-dimensional representation of a tai chi which is actually a sphere since the movement of yin and yang in the universe and humans occurs in three-dimensions.

The symbol shows the balance between yin and yang. A dark yin "fish" and light yang "fish" hugging one another represents a gradual rather than sudden change in balance between yin and yang. One increases as the other decreases. The small dark "eye" in the large light "fish" is yin in yang. Yin begins in yang when yang has reached its fullest extent. The small light "eye" in the large dark "fish" is yang in yin. Yang begins in yin when yin has reached its fullest extent. The S-curved line where the yin and yang "fish" join represents the line of life. This line is not straight because changes in yin and yang never happen in a straight line and the amounts of yin and yang are rarely equal. Just as the changes between yin and yang never happen in a straight line, life never happens in a straight line. People sometimes think a straight line in good because it is faster and direct, but life does not work that way. There are no short cuts to success in life.

The tai chi symbol also represents the river of time flowing within a timeless universe from when the universe was a spiral of gases into infinity. The light side of the symbol represents timelessness and the dark side symbolizes a universe that has no boundaries.

According to Chinese philosophy, before the universe existed there was only the absolute stillness of *Wuji* which is translated as Ultimateless or Boundless. Change began when *Wuji* gave rise to "the one" which is Tai Chi (*taiji*), the Supreme Ultimate. This Oneness is the Dao. The universe began when Tai Chi initiated movement which differentiated into "the two" which are yin and yang. The two became the four of "fish" of yin and yang and the "eyes" of yin in yang and yang in yin. The four became the eight which became the sixty-four which represents Ten Thousand Myriad Things (*wanwu*) which symbolizes the totality of everything in the Oneness that is the Dao. Flux in and among the Ten Thousand Myriad Things continues into infinity. This motion of the universe from the undifferentiated chaos that preceded the progression from Wuji to Ten Thousand Myriad Things is expressed in the deep meaning of the yin-yang symbol.

According to legend, the seeds of what became the Yijing (*I Ching*) were planted by Fu Xi (*Fuxi*), an ancient sage who developed a system of lines help people understand how to live with the rhythms of nature. His system, in which an unbroken line (   ) represents yang and a broken line (— —) represents yin, was applied to the same cosmology represented by the tai chi symbol. The two, yin and yang, became the four which were two yang lines, two yin lines, a yang line over a yin line, and a yin line over a yang line. One yang line or one yin line was added to each of the four to make eight trigrams or bagua. Ba means eight and gua is the word translated as trigram. The eight trigrams are ☰ Heaven (*qian*), ☷ Earth (*kun*), ☳ Thunder (*zhen*), ☶ Mountain (*gen*), ☱ Lake (*dui*), ☴ Wind (*xun*), ☵ Water (*kan*), and ☲ Fire (*li*). The eight trigrams were combined to form sixty-four hexagrams that became the basis of the *Yi Jing* (*I Ching*). Each six-line hexagram is made by combining two three-line trigrams placing them one above the other. Originally, *Yi Jing* contained only symbols that represented complex concepts. Later, words were added by King Wen (*Zhou Wen Wang*) who felt compelled to write descriptions of the natural rhythms depicted in *Yi Jing*. Confucius, also called Master Kong (*Kong Fuzi*), added information to the *Yi Jing* to make it easier to understand.

According to Shifu Cheng, the origins of tai chi chuan are rooted in the eight directions associated with these eight trigrams. Each trigram is associated with a manifestation of universe – heaven, earth, thunder, mountain, fire, water, lake, and wind. In addition, each trigram is associated with a direction and these are associated with corners and sides and Eight Gates in tai chi chuan. In addition to these external connections, many deep secrets about tai chi chuan are hidden within the *Yi Jing*.

Shifu taught, "There is heaven, other people, and yourself. You can control yourself, but not heaven or others. Follow the rhythms of nature and use the principles of *Yi Jing* to change yourself. Applying this philosophy can improve your life and improve your health. When yin gets to its fullest, yang starts. When yang gets to its fullest, yin starts. The changes may be large or small. Any time there is movement yin expands as yang contracts or yang expands as yin contracts. In your life journey do not rush to the end because when you arrive at a place of fullness, change will happen and your life will go in a different way. When you get to the top you begin to move toward the bottom. Once you reach your goal then you will start moving beyond it and lose the goal. Life is about the journey rather than achieving the goal."

3 STAGES OF LEARNING TAI CHI

Just as a map is a useful tool when undertaking a journey to a distant city, a guiding framework can be a useful tool on one's journey with tai chi. Each learner's journey with tai chi is different and each learner advances differently. Progress is spiraling and never-ending rather than a linear march through the stages. Tai chi practitioners continue to refine principles learned in earlier stages.

Stage 1 – Beginner

Beginners on learning the sequence of movements. Incorporating basic principles will help students build a strong foundation for future learning.

1. *Relax the mind* - Relax the mind before starting any tai chi form. The long-term goal is to be mentally relaxed yet focused on what you are doing throughout the entire form. Relaxing *xin*, often translated as heart-mind, becomes important after years of practice. Chinese understand xin (*xin*) as a synthesis of the emotions and the mind or consciousness. Two famous phrases

show the importance of a person's *xin*. One is *xiang you xin sheng* which means that which shows on one's face reflects one's actions and one's heart. The other is *jing you xin zhuan* which means one's view of and feelings about a situation are based on the status of the heart-mind/*xin*.

2. *Relax the body* - Relax the body before starting any tai chi form. Relax the body, but not so much that force is lost. The goal is to be physically relaxed yet focused throughout the entire form.

3. *Relax chest and round back* — Relaxing the shoulders relaxes the chest which allows the back to be slightly rounded. Pulling the shoulders back in the way a soldier stands at attention raises the chest. Raising the chest makes it difficult to sink qi to the dantian.

4. *Hold head and torso straight* - The head should be straight and neck relaxed. The torso is erect with the spine straight, but relaxed. Neither the head nor torso should bend or lean to the side, front, or back. Leaning forward, backward, or to the side rather than holding the body erect is a common mistake. Twisting the body to one side or the other when it should be facing forward is a common mistake usually caused by an error in the placement of the feet.

5. *Hold neck straight with chin drawn in* - Keeping the neck straight with chin gently drawn your chin has the dual functions of protecting the throat and pointing the crown of the head (*bai hui*) upward which allows qi to enter the body. The *bai hui* is located at the intersection of a line running up the nose and across top of head with line running across top of head from the point of one ear to point of the other ear. Bai means one hundred and *hui* means many things connect at one spot. *Bai hui* is the place where many major and minor meridians connect. Maintain a slightly drawn in chin throughout any tai chi form.

6. *Drop shoulders and elbows* - Dropping the shoulders allows them to relax which allows the body to relax which allows qi to sink to the lower dantian. Raised shoulders interfere with relaxation and causes qi to "float" rather than sinking to the dantian. Dropping the elbows so that they point downward rather than sideways contributes to relaxing the body.

7. *Sink qi to dantian* - Beginners simply imagine qi sinking to the dantian. The long-term goal is to learn to use your intention (*yi*) to sink qi to dantian.

8. *Align knees and toes* - There are multiple aspects of correct alignment of toes and knees. For correct alignment, imagine standing on a board with the foot is aligned with the board and

the knee is aligned with the board and foot. Allowing the knees to collapse inward is poor form and, over time, can damage knees. The ideal when bending the knee is to a line perpendicular to the floor from the tip of the toes, not the tip of the shoes. Stopping before the maximum point is acceptable, but extending beyond the toes stresses the knee and will cause damage over time.

9. *Use proper stepping technique* – Stepping wide enough yet not too wide contributes to stability. Steps are initiated by lifting the heel or toe, depending on the move. When stepping forward, the heel touches first. When stepping backwards or sideways, the toe touches first. Whether stepping forward, backward, or sideways the foot rolls to the floor gradually as weight is slowly transferred to it. Turning the foot is done either by lifting the toe and pivoting on the ball of the foot or lifting the ball of the foot and pivoting on the heel depending on the particular form. After turning the foot, adjusting it to the correct angle for each form is important to prevent knee damage.

10. *Shift weight correctly* - Shifting weight correctly is the first step in developing the rootedness that is the core of any style of tai chi. Learning proper shifting from the start builds good habits and avoids having to unlearn bad habits later. Shifting weight properly improves balance, promotes stability, and protects the

knees. The principle of shifting weight correctly is closely related to the principle of clearly differentiating full and empty which can be introduced once learners understand proper alignments.

11. *Clearly differentiate full and empty* - When shifting weight, clearly distinguish full and empty in the legs by "sitting down" on the back leg and allowing the foot of the front leg to lightly touch the ground. This principle is closely related to the principle of shifting weight correctly which focuses on understand proper alignments of feet, knees, legs, and hips. Understanding proper alignments is a precursor to differentiating full and empty.

Stage 2 – Advanced Beginner

Advanced beginners continue to focus on learning the sequence of movements as well as incorporating a few additional principles.

12. *Use proper hand position* - Tai Chi Palm requires keeping your palm relaxed and soft, fingers slightly separated, and your fingers and palm slightly curved. Form a Tai Chi Fist by keeping your knuckles from midpoint of fingers back to hand flat while keeping a space in the center of your fist so it is hollow.

13. *Pivot on axis of body* - Imagine a tent pole as the axis of the body. The body turns on this axis in the way the hub of a bicycle wheel turned on its side would turn on this axis.

14. *Turn waist* - In tai chi, waist refers to the hips (*kua*) and not the area a belt circles the torso (*yao*). Turn waist means pivoting your torso from your "tai chi waist" which is the hips, not the "belt waist." When turning the waist, imagine the hips and shoulders forming the corners of a rectangular plane. Turning from the tai chi waist promotes circulation within meridians. Turning the belt waist further than the hips is a common mistake. Turning the waist, the axis of all tai chi chuan movement, can generate a great deal of force. A more advanced understanding of the *kua* is developed in the next stage of learning.

Stage 3 – Intermediate

Intermediate students focus on refining the details of forms and postures learned previously. Learning additional principles is incorporated into the refining process.

15. *Open arm pits* - Having a small open space under the arm pits enables qi to flow easily. Holding arms close to body rather than open with a bit of space between the arm and body is a common mistake.

16. *Tuck tailbone* - Tucking the tailbone when performing tai chi forms improves the flow of qi in the meridians between the bottom of the spine (*wei lu* which is near the *hui yin* acupuncture point) and crown of the head (*niwan* which is near the *bai hui* acupuncture point).

17. *Open and relax the kua* - There is no English translation for *kua*. The *kua* is the area of the hip where the ball of the femur connects with the pelvis. Open and relax the *kua* by bending the knees and keeping knees opened outward with the hips dropped. Opening the knees aligns the knees with the toes. The *kua* is also an invisible energy gate which is related to the flow of qi.

18. *Maintain curves and circles* - All movements of tai chi reflect the curves of the tai chi symbol; there is no straight movement in tai chi. The largest curves are the circular movements in each form. Smaller curves and circles are in the movements of the hands and legs or the position of the arms. Smaller still is the curve in a relaxed palm. An internal energy known as *nei jing* spirals internally in a way that parallels the spiraling of the universe. Curved and circular movement improves internal circulation.

19. *Step lightly* - Transfer your weight slowly and lightly when you step forward, backward, or sideways. Imagine stepping lightly like a cat or walking on thin ice.

20. *Be soft and flexible* - Being soft is not the same as being relaxed. Being soft means having "tender tendons" that are as flexible and

limber as a dancer. Being soft allows qi to flow more effectively than when a body holds tension. The long-term goal is to become soft outside, but hard as steel inside.

21. *Maintain body height and posture* - Maintain a consistent height throughout any form. A common mistake is standing higher in some forms and lower with more bend in the knees in other forms. Although a lower form is desirable, it is more important to play at a level that can be maintained consistently. Eventually, the form can be done lower as leg strength builds over time.

22. *Be aware of opposites* - Full and empty, up and down, yin and yang are some of the opposites that co-exist in tai chi. Promoting the balance of yin and yang within the body by constantly shifting forward and backward, right and left, and up and down is a unique benefit of tai chi. The movements of tai chi silently convey the message that everything changes then balances, changes again and balances again over and over. Absorbing this message contributes to developing a calm, peaceful frame of mind.

Stage 4 – Advanced

Advanced tai chi practitioners begin to learn internal aspects of tai chi only after years of learning and practicing the external aspects of tai chi. Students work internally to strengthen *jing*, *qi*, and *shen* and to understand how to use intention and internal force (*jing*) together. The external aspects have significant physical and emotional health benefits; however, incorporating the external and internal aspects yield the greatest benefit.

23. *Synchronize all body movements* - All body parts move in unity. The movement of arms and legs are coordinated with each other and the rest of the body such as the turn of the head. The gaze the eyes is coordinated with the rest of the body.

24. *Strengthen jing, qi, and shen* –Playing tai chi improves *jing*, *qi*, and *shen* which translate as essence, energy, and spirit. Over time, *jing* becomes *qi*, *qi* becomes *shen*.

   a. Essence or *jing* is the root of life. *Jing* includes "being" substances that can be seen such as semen and "non-being" substances that cannot be seen. *Jing* maintains life activity and is responsible for reproduction, growth, development, and defense. This type of *jing* is vitality or life energy rather than *jing* or *jin* that is internal force. *Jing* is also the original energy (*yuan qi*) inherited from parents.

   b. *Qi* is the driving force of the universe, each living thing, and each human. *Qi* is a non-being substance that makes up everything in the universe. All material things result from the movement of *qi*. Without *qi* life could not exist. Moving slowly supports the ability to sense *qi* in the body. Beginners play tai chi slowly, however, advanced players strive to move more and more slowly. Slowing the pace automatically adds calmness.

    c. *Shen*, or spirit, is the governor of life. It includes intention, emotions, and knowledge as well as the soul and guides behaviors and actions and can be thought of as the leader of one's life. *Shen* can be seen as a flame in the eyes during tai chi.

25. *Use intention and jin together* - *Jin* (can be spelled *jing*) is a type of internal energy. Playing tai chi improves *jin* which, in turn, can lengthen life. Intention is used to control *jin*, *qi* controls your *jin* internally. An advanced student can have powerful *jin* yet may feel nothing. Tai chi chuan is a martial art that combines the hardness of steel with the softness of cotton and emphasizes use of intention rather than force or strength.

26. *Coordinate breathing and posture* – Once a person can be calm and relaxed when playing tai chi, she or he can learn to harmonize the breath. This means breathing deeply and imagining breathing to and from the dantian to bring qi to the dantian.

27. *Coordinate internal and external force* - Tai chi is unique since movement, intention, and *qi* harmonize the inside and outside of your body while most sports are external only. If you are relaxed your tendons become soft. Softness results in strength. You might look soft on the outside, but internally a tai chi player has

internal power (*jin*), agility (*ling*), and flexibility. If you strike someone it will have strength and agility.

28. *Incorporate eight types of force (ba jin)* - Grasp Peacock's Tail (*lǎn què wěi*) is a major form that includes four of the eight types of force – ward off (*peng*), roll back (*liu*), press (*ji*), and push (*an*). The others are pull-down (*cai*), split (*lie*), elbow stroke (*zhou*), and shoulder stroke (*kao*). The eight types of force are sometimes called the Eight Gates (*bā mén*) which are associated with the eight directions.

29. *Move like a river or cloud* - In beginning stages of learning tai chi, moving like a river means shifting the body evenly and steadily through all tai chi forms without pauses. It is important to fully complete each form with a split second between that feels like a pause even though it is so brief as to be almost non-existent. The feet never stop although the palms may stop. In the intermediate stage, moving like a river refers to moving *qi* evenly and steadily inside the body. The highest level of tai chi is to have no body form, no substance. The whole body is empty. Everything is forgotten. Even a tiger or dragon screaming does not result in distraction. The peacefulness of flowing water or a cloud permeates all.

4 TAI CHI SALUTE

The tai chi salute carries multiple layers of meaning. The most
obvious meaning is the gesture of respect shown to one's teacher or
an opponent when the salute is performed at the beginning and end
of each round of tai chi. The tai chi salute is executed by touching the
open, flat palm of the left hand to the right fist with arms held in a
circle at shoulder height. The right hand is held so that the "eye" of
the side of the fist faces outward. The curved left thumb fits in the
hole made by the thumb and curled fingers of the right hand. In
class or practice at home, the salute is executed standing still with feet
parallel. When giving a tai chi demonstration, the salute is initiated
by stepping forward on the right foot and lifting the arms into a circle
as the left foot is moving toward the right foot. The salute is
completed as the left foot is placed next to the right foot.

The salute is a pledge to live by two important concepts. The first is
symbolized by circled arms represent holding the entire world to

communicate "*si hai yi jia*" which translates as "four seas, one family." It means that no matter how different people are and how far apart we live, all people are one family. Each member of a tai chi community is expected to act in ways that promote justice and the greatest good of all – self, family, country, and the world. The left thumb tucked into the hole made by the thumb and curled fingers of the right hand represents the expectation of acting with humility.

The second concept is symbolized by the left hand covering the right fist to communicate "*wen wu he yi*" which translates as "culture and martial arts synthesized into one." The right fist represents the physical power of martial arts (*wu*) and the left palm represents the civility of culture (*wen*). Physical power unfettered by civility can result in brutality. Culture lacking physical power cannot bring positive intention to fruition. Physical power balanced with and fused to civility contributes to what Daoists call integrity or inner power and what Confucians call moral character or virtue.

The deepest layer of meaning is the fingers representing the five virtues that are the foundation of Confucian ethics. The thumb represents benevolence, index finger represents morality, middle finger represents propriety, ring finger represents knowledge and wisdom, and the pinky represents honesty. These virtues are interlinked and each strengthens the others.

Benevolence (*Ren*)

Benevolence, which means having a loving and caring heart, is the most basic and important of the five Confucian virtues. It is demonstrated by treating people, animals, and the earth with equal kindness just as the sun shines on everything without favoring any person, animal, or place on earth. Benevolence can be practiced in a tai chi community that parallels the structure of a family. The teacher is treated with the respect given to one's parents, senior students are esteemed as older siblings, and new students are guided and encouraged as younger sisters and brothers.

Morality (*Yì*)

Morality is the fabric in which the Confucian virtues are woven together. Although often translated as righteousness, it is better understood as the moral obligation to do the right thing for the right reason, to fulfill one's duties, and to act with fairness, honor, loyalty, generosity, and charity. Each member of a tai chi community is responsible for carefully discerning what is right and fair then acting for the greatest good of all concerned.

Propriety (*Li*)

Propriety, which means doing the right thing at the right time, focuses on promoting harmony on both personal and societal levels. Propriety on a personal level is demonstrated by respect for self and others and by behaving with self-control, appropriate etiquette, and courtesy which results in harmonious relationships with others. Propriety on the societal level can refer to a well-ordered natural flow as in the flow of the four seasons or a well-ordered society that functions with good political order. Individuals contribute at the social level by conforming to societal norms and respecting the government.

Knowledge and Wisdom (*Zhi*)

Zhi is particularly difficult to translate since it carries a complex, dual meaning. Young people use their minds to amass as much conceptual knowledge as possible. They also acquire social knowledge about how to act with benevolence, morality, and propriety; however, their actions can be hollow because youth have not lived long enough to develop moral wisdom. Over time, through sincere practice and study, moral wisdom develops internally which enables an individual to know right from wrong and to differentiate good from evil. Mature people use their accumulated wisdom to act with integrity, tolerance, flexibility, and good judgment to promote interpersonal harmony.

Honesty *(Xìn)*

Honesty incorporates acting with integrity and being trustworthy. Meaning what you say and doing what you say you will do is the key to gaining the trust of others. Honesty strengthens all virtues because it is about keeping one's words and actions. There is a Confucian saying, "There is no place for a person to stand if he does not have honesty."

5 TAIJI ORGANS

In Chinese thought, there are two fundamental categories of the universe – non-being (*wu*) and being (*you*). Non-being is understood as that which cannot be seen and being is that which can be seen. For example, meridians are as real as blood vessels; however, meridians cannot be seen so they are non-being while blood vessels can be seen and are being. It is important to note that the metaphysical association of non-being with spirit that is typical in western thought is absent in Chinese thought.

Ancient people determined these categories using physical eyes and the Eye of Heaven (*tian yian*) located between the eyebrows. Physical eyes can see only one-third of the universe that is being while the two-thirds that is non-being can be seen only by using the eye of heaven. Sensing or seeing with the Eye of Heaven is known as internal proof or internal confirmation (*nei zheng*).

The human body is a small universe that parallels the natural universe so it also contains non-being (*wu*) and being (*you*). Internal proof is the basis of traditional Chinese medicine. Internal proof seen with the Eye of Heaven was used to understand the internal structure of the human body. Ancients using internal proof could see the energy flow among internal organs. They observed humans and determined how disease begins and how to cure it. Internal proof was confirmed via external proof by observing symptoms over thousands of years. Over many centuries, Chinese physicians developed the knowledge that disease can be cured by changing emotions which, in turn, changes and heals the physical body.

People used internal proof to see that the human body contains invisible, non-being taiji organs. There is no English translation of taiji organs. Taiji organs are spheres that are like the taiji symbol (*taiji tu*) when it is thought of as three-dimensional. Each has yin and yang. Sometimes they are like light and sometimes they are like qi. Some are about the size of a mung bean while others are large. Major taiji organs are the three dantians – upper (*yin tang*), middle (*dan zhong*), and lower (*dantian*). Many tai chi organs are concentrated in acupuncture points such as the palm *lao gong*, foot bubbling well (*yong quan*), *bai hui* in crown of head. Each taiji organ is a holograph of the entire universe.

Taiji organs in your body are important yet western physicians are unaware of them because they exist in the realm of non-being. Taiji organs control the five internal organs and the organs that correspond to them. Taiji organs function to receive energy then release it. They also organize and regulate energy so that life can continue. Taiji organs are constantly turning and stoppage occurs only if there is a problem in the body. If there is a problem in these organs illness can develop. Taiji organs can become medicine for up to two days and assist in the process of rebalancing yin and yang and releasing bad energy.

According to Daoist philosophy, playing the tai chi chuan Yang Style Long Form just once exercises all the taiji organs in your body. This happens automatically with no thought or effort on the part of the tai chi chuan player.

6 EIGHT GATES AND FIVE STEPS

Although Shifu Cheng asserted that the Five Steps and Eight Gates are important in tai chi and implied they are involved in the three phases of tai chi practice (first, understand conscious movement, second, interpret energy, and third, spiritual illumination) she simply named the eight gates and the directions with which they are associated. She also taught that the feet step out the Five Steps which allows control of the eight directions. The Five Steps are related to the Five Elements. She promised to teach her disciples more, but died before doing so.

The eight gates are:

1. Ward Off – peng – south
2. Roll Back – liu – west
3. Press – ji – east
4. Push – an – north

5. Pull down – cai – northwest
6. Split – lie – southeast
7. Elbow stroke – zhou – northeast
8. Shoulder stroke – kao – southwest

The five steps are:

1. Advance – jin bu – Fire
2. Retreat – tui bu – Water
3. Gaze Left – zuo gu – Wood
4. Look Right – you pan – Metal
5. Central Equilibrium – Zhong ding – Earth

Translating the concept of Five Elements (*wu xing*) from Chinese to English is difficult. Although the English word element is the closest translation for the Chinese word *xing*, element in English represents something that is stagnant or motionless. In reality, the Five Elements are dynamic and constantly moving. Translating five elements as five phases or five elemental phases is used more and more frequently in modern translations of Chinese texts since these phrases imply movement.

7 ZHAN ZHUANG VERSUS MA BU

Shifu allowed students to choose between practicing Zhan Zhuang or Ma Bu during standing practice in class. What is the difference between the two?

ZHAN ZHUANG / STANDING STAKE

A form of qigong that heals and improves the entire body. It can be done outside everyday as long as it is not windy and the head is kept warm. *Zhan zhuang* should be performed for at least twenty minutes and no more than an hour.

To perform *zhan zhuang* start with your feet together then side step to shoulder width apart. Open your crotch to a half circle then bend your knees a little. Keep your hips down. The open crotch and hips down opens circulation in the *ren mai*. Your head is held straight with the tongue touching the top of the mouth. Drop your elbows and shoulders. *Zhan zhuang* has three important circles – open crotch, arms, and hands with fingers pointing towards each other.

Breathing is important in *zhan zhuang*. Start breathing naturally then gradually shift to abdominal breathing. Image a small ball contracts slightly as you inhale and expands slightly as you exhale.

MA BU / HORSE STANCE

A leg strengthening exercise that supplements tai chi chuan. Your feet are wider than shoulder width. Over time, deepen your stance by trying one minute at a lower stance and increase the length of time you can stand in a low stance until you are able to bend legs as deeply as possible throughout your ma bu practice. Open crotch. Raise hands to shoulder level and make a circle with fingers pointing to each other.

At end, bring palms to sides and in front of body with palms facing downward then close by bringing feet together and standing up.

Relax!

8 TYPES OF QIGONG

There are four main types of qigong – Daoist, Buddhist, Confucian, and healing. Daoists and Buddhists both hold that the true nature of humans is pure; however, it becomes contaminated by human problems. Both seek a state of non-being and returning original spirit (*yuanshen*) results in happiness, having lots of qi, and enlightenment; however, their approaches to qigong are different. Daoists believe essence (*jing*) becomes energy (*qi*) which becomes spirit (*shen*) which becomes *xu* which is emptiness or void. Xu is the same as the non-being that is sought by Buddhists.

Daoist qigong is health oriented and uses techniques that cultivate mind, heart, and body. The purposes are to promote long life, connect the mind and body, and cultivate virtue. Buddhist meditation is spiritual. Buddhist practices involve mind, heart, and spirit. The body is unimportant. Buddhist meditation is very simple - no thinking. Confucian qigong is a middle way that utilizes some technique and some intent to cultivate virtue and to create balance and harmony in heart and mind. Healing qigong promotes health in the short term and cultivates virtue done over the long-term. There are types of qigong to heal specific illnesses.

There are two categories of qigong within the four types. *Jin gong* involves calmly sitting or standing as in *zhan zhuang*. *Dong gong* requires slow movement coordinated with breathing as in *le gong*. Tai chi chuan when done quite slowly is a kind of *dong gong*.

Any type of qigong is a treasure that improves health. People have different needs that are the result of a combination of genes, life experience, and the physical environment. Each person has unique needs, gifts, and potentials. Qigong is a golden key that unlocks the potentials in an individual.

The body has a special kind of qi during qigong. You might experience it as a sensation of coldness, itchiness, swelling, heat, or numbness. These sensations are all positive signs. Qi during qigong is like a large amount of water flowing through an area and breaking through blockages so that circulation can improve. You might experience pain in a particular area of your body because special qi is healing your body or is healing a future disease and preventing it from a current.

9 HAPPY HEART QIGONG/LE XIN GONG

Happy Heart Qigong/*Le Xin Gong* was developed by Shifu Cheng to promote calmness and self-healing via a synthesis of traditional Daoist and Buddhist techniques and philosophy. Shifu Cheng taught students primarily by doing this qigong. The information in this chapter is a synthesis of bits of information spoken in response to student questions. This chapter is presented in words as close as possible to her own words.

TECHNIQUE FOR HAPPY HEART QIGONG

The goal is to do qigong daily throughout your whole life. Daily qigong is particularly important if you have a health issue since daily practice is the most effective for strengthening your immunity. If you are ill it is desirable to increase your practice time beyond what you do normally. The more you do qigong the more useful it is.

Happy Heart Qigong/*Le Xin Gong* can be practiced indoors or outdoors. For indoor practice select a quiet place where you will not be disturbed. The room should be warm or you should wear enough clothes to be warm. It is best to practice in the same room every time you do qigong because it will gradually build a residual energy field that will support your practice. Outdoor practice is good. Practicing near moving water is good because of the negative ions near water. Near a lake is better than a river because it is calmer. Practicing near the ocean is okay, but not as good as lake or river. Avoid outdoor practice on a rainy or windy day or if mosquitoes are biting.

You can sit on the floor with legs crossed or in a chair, but not on a bed because the softness makes it difficult to be relaxed while you hold your body straight. Sitting on a pillow on the floor concentrates the energy circulation the torso. Sitting in a chair lengthens the path of energy circulation since it must pass through legs. It takes a long time to shift to being able to sit on the floor for qigong without your legs falling asleep. Whether you sit on the floor or in a chair it is best if your legs are open rather than close together because open enables energy to flow easily. If you sit on the floor, sitting in the lotus position is preferable to simply crossing your legs. It is important to sit on a pillow or cushion that prevents coldness from the floor seeping into your body. Remove your shoes if you sit on the floor. Women place their right leg on top and men the left leg on top. If you sit on a chair, sit forward on the edge of the chair to allow energy flow around your body. Do not lean against the back of the chair because it is easier on your spine and kidney meridians and *dumai* and blocks circulation. Select a chair that allows you to sit with your legs at ninety-degree angle with feet flat on the floor. The chair should be firm. Keep your shoes on so that coldness does not enter your body through the soles of your feet.

The starting position for your hands is in front of your dantian with palms slightly curved and facing upward. Palms are a few inches apart and relaxed. Women place right hand above the left, men place left hand above right. This starting position is best for starting qi flow in your body during qigong. Once started, the qi flow generated during the qigong may move your hands into a different position. Allow your body to move if movement happens on its own, but do not consciously move your body except to return to the starting position once your body calms.

There are a few important considerations for doing qigong. Cover your legs and feet with a blanket whether you sit on the floor on in a chair. There are important pressure points on the legs and it is particularly easy for coldness to enter these points when you are relaxed. It is okay to have the blanket around your whole body, although the main reason is for feet and legs. Wait for at least twenty to thirty minutes after eating to begin your practice. An hour is better. Not eating means there is no food in the stomach. Qigong can help circulation in the stomach meridian. Wear loose fitting clothes. Do not wear a hat, belt, or watch during qigong because they interfere with circulation of blood and qi. Remove your eyeglasses and watch before beginning qigong. Use the bathroom before beginning qigong. If you need to urinate or have a bowel movement during qigong get up and use the bathroom without waiting for qigong to end. Return to qigong when done in the bathroom.

Doing qigong the same time each day is best because your body will become used to the routine, but regardless of the time of day doing qigong daily is better than not doing it. Doing qigong in the early morning can be helpful in having good energy for the day. Practice before eating breakfast. Doing qigong before you go to sleep at night is very good. Sleeping after qigong is different than regular sleep.

STAGES OF HAPPY HEART QIGONG

Happy Heart Qigong is a sitting qigong with three stages: 1) Adjust body/*tiao shen* in which your posture and body are adjusted by relaxing. It is relatively easy. 2) Adjust qi/*tiao qi* in which qi is adjusted through breathing. This harder to do. The goal is to have abdominal breathing begin naturally. 3) Adjust spirit or intention/*tiao xin*. *Xin* is often translated heart-mind, but has no equivalent in English and can best be understood as a synthesis of emotions and consciousness. The nervous system is also adjusted in this part of qigong. This stage is difficult and takes a long time to develop.

Stage 1 – Adjust Body

When you do qigong relax first, be calm second, and follow nature third. Relax your body as you maintain a straight posture with the intention to allow qi from nature to enter your head. Relaxing your body does not mean letting your body fall over. It means relaxing internally. Relax your spirit. Have an open heart. Be optimistic. Dropping your shoulders, relaxing your chest, and slightly rounding your back opens the spine for easy circulation so your qi can clear. Calmness is the core of doing qigong. It is the only thing that is necessary during qigong. The amount of calmness varies from day to day, but any time you are calm it is good for your body. Calmness during the adjust body/*tiao shen* phase of qigong calms you internally. Your mind can become calm like water on a lake. Chang San Feng, the founder of tai chi chuan, did qigong in wind and rain and was still able to stay calm. Sometimes qi will move your body. Follow it and allow it to happen. Do not direct the body to move, just follow it. Not moving during qigong is fine. Maybe your body is already strong and healing movement is not needed. Follow nature during qigong. Follow it in all of your life.

There are several signs that you are receiving qi during qigong. Your whole body might feel calm and relaxed or have a sense of heaviness. Breathing will be slow and thin. Your mind is focused with fewer and fewer thoughts. Your skin might itch, have a feeling of electricity, or twitching of an area on the surface of the skin. You might experience numbness that is not the numbness of sitting a long time or heat in either the entire body or a part of the body. If you do not experience these signs do not pursue them. Follow what is natural for you. Desires during qigong are not helpful so let go of what you want. Do not think about what you want to happen and try to make it happen. Instead, follow what is natural in the moment and allow qi to move naturally in your body. The more you let go of daily experience and the more you take an expanded view rather than dwelling of difficulties the more qi you can receive. Disturbed emotion in daily life makes it more difficult to be calm during qigong. If there is something difficult happening in your life try to keep your mind off it at least for some of the time during qigong. Remember that things happen in life. Analyze what you can do and do it. Then, let it go instead of talking about it and worrying about it day after day.

It is important to be calm and relaxed throughout qigong because it is possible to receive more good energy when you're relaxed. Practice calmness and you can receive everything. In the Adjust Body Stage, relax your body by consciously letting go of the tension in each part of your body starting with the head and moving toward the toes. Focus your attention on your lower dantian. Each student should watch her own body. Over time, practice gradually trains you to focus and to relax.

Stage 2 – Adjust Breathing

It is important to use correct breathing technique when doing qigong.

Qi can be understood as breath or energy. Gong means time and practice. Understanding qi is very important, however, there is no English word for qi. Energy is a word that is often used, but it is not adequate. Qi allows the universe to exist and movement to occur in the universe. Your body is a small universe that contains the same qi as the universe. Without qi the world would not be able to live and there would be no circulation in your body.

Breathing properly is very important because qigong breathing is different from regular breathing. Qigong is healing because it regulates the movement of qi. – qi is yang, yin is in blood. Qigong breathing "softens" blood and relaxes the body which improves circulation within the body and within meridians. The movement of qi heals current illnesses and prevents future illness because it moves stagnation away before it has a physical effect.

At first, breathe in whatever way is natural for you. Breathing in a relaxed and comfortable way without attempting to control your breath will create calmness. Later, use your intention to breathe long, deeply, and thinly with longer pauses then your breathing to strengthen the lungs, diaphragm, dantian and to balance yin and yang. Thin breathing is like drawing a silk string to the dantian. Breathing with that intention will gradually develop the proper technique over time. Cultivate the ability to breathe this way with comfort and a relaxed feeling. Breathing with just with the lungs is not deep so when your practice is more advanced try abdominal breathing at least some of the time during qigong. If you do not intentionally control breathing then you will not develop the longer breath. If you do not use your intention, your breathing will improve, but you will never get to the most effective long, slow breathing. To do deeper in qigong you should think about controlling your breathing sometimes, but not constantly. Guiding breath with your mind will eventually result in deeper breathing naturally.

All bodies are different so some people have a harder time learning the different types of breathing. Relaxed breathing is the key regardless of the type you do. When you are learning qigong breathing it is important to not worry about what how you're breathing. If you are calm, you will be fine. If you force the wrong type of breathing it can do harm. Let your body control how you breathe.

There are over twenty types of qigong breathing that have varied lengths for inhaling and exhaling. The basic technique for sitting qigong is to inhale by expanding your abdomen and using your intention to guide qi to your dantian. Do not think about breathing through your nose. It is important to inhale with the tongue touching the top of your mouth. Breathe smoothly, slowly, and naturally regardless of the length of your inhalation or exhalation. For each inhalation and exhalation do not breathe to the fullest possible amount of air taken into or expelled from the lungs. Instead of breathing from 0 – 100 breathe from 10-90. There should be a short pause just before you complete each inhale and at the end of each exhale. Over time the pauses should become longer. The breath should gradually become so soft that it would not move a feather.

When doing qigong at home, first breathe regularly and relaxed. Second, breathe thinly, deeply, evenly, and long. Third, as you feel stronger over time inhale to the mingmen/door of life starting with three times and gradually increase to nine times. Whatever you do, relax and follow what is natural for you on that day. Eventually this will help the qi flow in your meridians.

No thinking is best when you are focused on breathing although it is okay to think good energy is coming into your body when inhaling. It is also okay to think briefly of cells opening to good energy, a lotus flower blooming, or light entering the top of your head. The key is that if you follow what is natural for you, you will receive a lot of good energy through qigong breathing.

Stage 3 – Adjust Spirit

Shifu did not give verbal instruction about the third stage of Happy Heart Qigong. She frequently spoke about two topics that apply to all three stages of this qigong – avoiding thinking and controlling emotions. There are different levels of thinking during qigong. Absence of thinking is the most desirable level because you are one with the universe, however, not thinking is difficult to achieve. Thinking briefly of something beautiful such as a lotus, green trees, light from the sun, flowing water, the ocean, lakes, or mountains can help you be calm. Observing your mind chatter is better than uncontrolled chatter because it is progress from being in the chatter, but it is not as good not having chatter. It is acceptable to be aware of your internal experience. Allow yourself to experience whatever happens and avoid thinking about it. Afterward, it is okay to write about what happened and try to make sense of it. Do not think about deep theory during qigong, however, studying afterward is fine.

Thinking during qigong happens to everyone. Some people can relax and become calm quickly while others have a difficult time calming the mind. A beginner has more thoughts than a more experienced person so beginners must focus on not thinking. If you do qigong daily, some days you will be calm and some days your mind will be active. If your mind is active, control it. Having the intention to drop qi to your dantian can help. Thinking of something beautiful like a flower can help. Regardless of how you accomplish it, you must stop an active mind. Over time, this automatically leads to less thinking and periods of not thinking will lengthen.

When thoughts arise follow what is natural for you because trying hard not to think can result in tension. If you do think during qigong think positively. If a negative thought comes during qigong open your eyes and puff out the thought then return to meditation. If a pain or other physical sensation arises think "It's healing me" and don't worry since pain is simply pain. Techniques that can help calm your mind such as focusing on breathing thinly and deeply to shift the moment, sinking your mind to your dantian focusing on one thought or on my voice, or thinking of me supporting you.

Gradually, wisdom develops during qigong and answers to problems and questions come because intuition is inspired. Therefore, the more you do qigong the more okay it is to follow thoughts. It is acceptable for advanced students to focus on a problem if one arises during meditation.

Experiencing emotions during qigong is common and is part of the process of bringing emotions into balance. Each person is different and each experiences emotions at different times. Every time you do qigong it is different even if you're in the same environment. If you do qigong every day it is good regardless of what happens. You receive good energy every time you do qigong although the amount varies – sometimes a lot, sometimes a little. Regardless of what you experience your intent should be to stay calm no matter what emotions arise. It is advisable to calm down before beginning qigong if you are upset and to avoid beginning qigong if you are angry.

It is expected that emotions will emerge during qigong. If sadness, fear, or anger emerge during qigong it does not matter. Feel your feelings and continue qigong. Feeling these emotions during qigong can help release them from your body rather than letting them accumulate. Tears during meditation are very good because bad energy goes out with the tears so if you cry today then maybe you will feel better tomorrow. If you feel sad it can help if you think about light or think about your god supporting you. If you feel angry during qigong feel it rather than trying to control it because it can help the bad energy go out of your body. If you feel afraid during qigong, open your eyes and think once that Shifu is sending good energy then close your eyes and continue qigong. If a disturbing thought or image emerges while you are doing qigong, open your eyes and blow a puff of air from your mouth to blow the disturbance away. Too much emotion of any sort results in too much internal movement and this weakens the heart. You need to control yourself. Even too much happiness during qigong is not helpful. If you are too happy during qigong, notice the happiness, but try to calm yourself.

Doing qigong will help you become more peaceful and stable over time. Your temperament will gradually change so that you will worry or feel anger or sadness less frequently. More and more your body and emotions will be calm and unworried. Do not expect to see the results of qigong quickly. It must build gradually. If you do qigong daily it builds gradually, but if you skip days you lose some of what you have gained. If you are not moving forward you are moving backward.

DOING HAPPY HEART QIGONG/ LE XIN GONG

As her students know, Shifu taught this qigong by giving instructions throughout the forty-five minutes needed to complete the practice. Music composed and sung by her qigong master, Grandmaster Kong Tai, who had an ability of healing through the vibrations created as he sang. Master Kong arranged songs to support gradual deepening as students moved through the stages of Le Xin Gong. This section includes a list of the verbal instructions Shifu Cheng gave when leading Le Xin Gong integrated with details given in response to students asked questions after qigong. It is intended as a refresher for former students. It is impossible to learn how to do this particular qigong from the information in this section.

Stage 1 – Adjust Body/Tiao Shen
1. Close your eyes and keep them closed throughout qigong.
2. Head straight with the top pointing upward, draw in your chin slightly. This allows the *beihuei* to point upward to receive qi from the heavens and qi can move inside you. *Beihuei* and *hueiyin* should be in a line to assist qi flow.

3. Close your mouth.

4. Tongue touching top of mouth - Tongue touching top of mouth is important. Closed mouth with tongue touching the palate, teeth not together. It is best to keep your tongue on the top of your mouth throughout qigong, however, each person has a different way of holding their jaws and teeth so for the rest of the mouth do whatever is natural for you. Tongue touching palate the whole time we are doing qigong is desirable, but doing what is natural is most important. Hold mouth naturally.

5. Look at the tip of your nose once - Some people experience movement of their eyes during qigong. If this occurs, focus your attention on your dantian. Do not control the movement of your eyes.

6. Smile gently - There is a very important spot just above the center of the lip and below the nose that is stimulated when a person smiles. This spot is called the *ren zhong* and is where the *ren mai* meridian down the front of your body and *du mai* meridian that runs up your back and across the top of your head come together. Stimulating that spot is important for long life. Relaxing the corners of the mouth is actually a way to smile gently and have the face be relaxed. There is no limitation to the length of time you smile as long as you remain relaxed.

7. Gently draw in your chin. This allows the *bai hui* to point upward to receive qi from the heavens and qi can move inside you. *Bai hui* and *huei yin* (located between genitals and anus) should be in a line to assist qi flow. There is a pressure point called the *bai hui* at

the top of the head. Regardless of the angle at which you hold yourself think of light energy showering down on you and swirling all around you.

8. Keep your spine and neck straight, but relaxed. This promotes circulation especially in the *du mai* meridian in your spine.

9. Waist straight, but relaxed

10. Draw in your abdomen

11. Draw in perineum for a short time. Gently lifting the perineum helps your energy. Drawing in abdomen and perineum at time of exhalation stores energy inside you. Using your intention to draw in the perineum once or twice supports circulation in the *ren mai* and *du mai* meridians. The *ren mai* meridian is in the front of the body and *du mai* meridian is in the back of the body. Having the tongue touching the top of the mouth while drawing in the perineum creates a connection between these two meridians. Drawing in the perineum also helps store *shen chi*.

12. Relax your chest and make your back round.

13. Drop your shoulders.

14. Open armpits. This allows energy circulation within arms and shoulders.

15. Relax your head

16. Relax your eyes

17. Relax your ears

18. Relax your nose

19. Relax your face

20. Relax your whole body again

21. Relax your chest

22. Relax your shoulders

23. Relax your arms

24. Relax your hands

25. Relax your fingers

26. Relax your whole body again

27. Relax your head

28. Relax your chest

29. Relax your hips

30. Relax your legs

31. Relax your toes

Stage 2 – Adjust Qi/Tiao Qi

1. Breathe thinly and deeply, evenly and long. When inhaling, the tongue touches the top of mouth. Inhaling thinly is the opposite of thick. It must be very slow to be thin. A fast inhale would bring in too much at one time and would be the thick. Try to make your breathing as thin as a silk thread. Breathing deeply means that when inhaling the qi comes in through the nose and intention is used to move it to the dantian. It is not with the lungs and chest. Evenly refers to keeping the intake of air consistent throughout the inhale rather than keeping the length of inhale and exhale even. Each person has different needs and the length of inhale and exhale changes accordingly so follow what is natural for you rather than trying to control your breath.

This might vary from day to day. A long inhale can be helpful if your digestion is not good or if your hands and feet are cold. A long exhale can be helpful if you have a headache, an eye problem, high blood pressure, or abdominal gas.

Once you have learned to relax begin learning abdominal breathing. Inhale by using your intention to expand the abdomen. This causes qi to go to the dantian. Inhaled good qi from the outside is combined with original qi/yuan qi. The xiao jiao/lower part of sanjiao holds original qi/yuan qi. Over time, abdominal breathing will become natural and will not require thought. Upon exhaling qi goes down the *ren mai* which helps qi accumulate in the dantian. Accumulating qi in the dantian is very important. Many meridians cross the dantian either directly or indirectly. Each is like a river coming to the dantian which is called *qi hai*/qi ocean.

2. Hold time. There is a slight pause at the end of inhale or exhale. Over time, the pause lengthens. The brief pause or "hold time" at the end of inhale is mostly commonly called *bi qi* in Chinese. Some people pause after the exhale. This is fine and could be due to a need to release bad qi. You should not count during hold time. Consciously do this technique for only a short time because doing it for too long builds tension within you. Remember to have your tongue touching the top of your mouth during hold time. Students are to breathe naturally most of the time and also practice holding the breath for a short time during

qigong. There is a brief pause between inhaling and exhaling. Be natural. Do not emphasize the pause, it is just a brief wait.

3. Exhale thinly and deeply, not to the end. Pause briefly before beginning to inhale. Not to the end means breathe not all the way in and not all the way out. If you exhale or inhale completely then you cannot relax. There is a slight pause at the end of inhale or exhale. Over time, the pause lengthens. Beginners should not attempt to the pause and experienced people practice having a comfortable pause. When exhaling the tongue can touch the top of mouth or drop down.

Stage 3 - Adjust spirit or intention/ *tiao xin*

1. Imagine your dantian feeling hot. Feel the warmth.
2. Imagine energy moving from *mingmen* to *dantian* three times. The *mingmen* (door of life) is the area low on the back where a fetus is initially joined to its mother via the umbilical cord. The mingmen is a major pressure point. Fetuses develop the mingmen first then kidneys second. After qigong your mingmen might be hot to the touch. If it is cold to the touch it means body energy is going out. If that happens you should do additional qigong to support the bad energy flowing out. Qi is adjusting you during regardless of what you sense.
3. Swallow saliva and send it to your dantian.
4. Imagine a lotus opening slowly in your dantian. This brings good energy into your dantian. Visualize the lotus during qigong

because this flower is very holy. Lotus grows from mud it symbolizes that a beautiful person can grow from a bad environment. Thinking lotus and bright light is very pure, calming. The flower is beautiful and the root and seeds are nutritious.

5. Imagine a lotus closing slowly in your dantian then think of nothing. Good energy enters body upon inhalation, spreads throughout body on exhale

6. Repeat the opening/closing of lotus a few times.

7. Clear your liver while imagining a green color. Do not worry about the colors and internal organs that are named in class. Thinking does not matter. Being calm and relaxed matters. It is better to imagine brighter shades rather than darker.

8. Clear your heart while imagining a red color

9. Clear your spleen while imagining a yellow color

10. Clear your lungs while imagining a white color. Think - your lungs are very pure.

11. Clear your kidneys while imagining a black color (imagining blue is acceptable)

12. Imagine your whole body being one with Light

13. Imagine your whole body being one with the Universe

14. Imagine your whole body being one with Nature

15. Imagine your body becoming smaller and smaller until you are totally empty. Your body can become very small or very big. Both mean your body is joining with the Universe. We expand and join the Universe or we get smaller and smaller until we join

the Universe. Either is joining with the Universe. That is the goal of qigong. Your Self expands into the Universe and you become the Universe. When your Self becomes smaller you remain as the Universe. Your Self disappears because the Self is so full of the Universe. The Universe is a combination of yin and ang. Doing qigong and tai ji balances yin and yang because you are flowing with the energy and laws of the Universe. If you continue practicing daily over a long period of time you will gradually understand more and more. You expand into Universe, become the Universe then when you become smaller you stay the Universe. You disappear because you are so full of Universe. As you practice qigong over time, you'll gradually understand more and more. If you go with the energy of the Universe and laws of the Universe then you will be in balance, your yin/yang will be balanced.

Closing

1. Swallow saliva and for one special time imagine it going to your dantian. During qigong the quality of saliva changes. It is a different type of saliva than during the rest of the day. It is useful for prolonging life.

2. Pull a ball of good energy by slowly moving hands together and apart at the level of the heart. Doing qigong generates lots of good energy. The motions of pushing and pulling help move the energy that has been generated. Horizontal pulling increases

good energy. It is important that the hands are horizontal at the level of the heart. Vertical pulling is for the heart. It is okay to do the hand motions any time, however, immediately after qigong is best. It is important that the hands are horizontal at the level of the heart. The way you breathe depends on what your body needs. Beginners can think of inhaling when opening hands, exhaling when pressing hands together, however, the timing of inhaling and exhaling when pulling energy does not matter.

Eventually, your abdomen will start abdominal breathing by itself. In the meantime, it is okay to do it consciously a little bit.

3. Press palms together at the middle dantian and think of the cells of body closing. Palms are pressed together at the level of the middle dantian. The heel of the palms where there is a crease/dent presses the middle dantian. This creates a connection from the hands to middle dantian as you are thinking closing. This is a very complex area. Inside the middle dantian is a small, hollow space called the can wang ting kung. It means palace. Kung means collective area. The dan zhong is a pressure point close to the location of the middle dantian. The two are different. Similarly, the upper dantian is inside the head in the area of what Hindus call the Third Eye while on the outside of that area there is a pressure point. Knowledge of the concept of meridians was developed by Daoist masters who could see inside the human body. This component of the closing is the only part of the closing motions that is not optional. It is crucial because not closing properly can cause loss of qi becomes your cells are

open from qigong. The cells are open during qigong and the other massages close the cells. The intention of closing the cells of the body is important. Not thinking too much is also important.

4. Closing in other forms of qigong. For standing qigong as well as five elements/wu xin and standing kidney qigong the closing is palms together, rub hands together then place hands over dantian.

5. Self-massage performed at the end of Happy Heart Qigong is described in the following chapter.

10 MARROW WASHING/XI SUI ZHEN JING

One's hands are particularly full of qi after practicing Happy Heart Qigong so it is an optimum time to do self-massage called Marrow Washing. It is important to do self-massage after qigong seriously since each movement has a purpose. As in the previous chapter, explanatory information after naming the technique was gleaned from answers to students' questions after qigong.

1. Rub palms together several times. Friction between the palms activates qi.

2. Click teeth together 36 times then run your tongue along the front of your teeth clockwise, then counterclockwise (at least nine times, thirty-six is better). Daoists developed internal exercises. Internal movements are more important than external movements. Qigong is an internal exercise rather than the external exercise of sports. Internal exercise clears cells and makes them healthier. There is an internal

connection between the tongue and heart (also nose and lungs) so moving the tongue helps the heart. Tongue circling teeth is good for spleen. Spleen is sensitive to damp. If spleen has dampness it creates lung mucus.

3. Massage face starting with palms on center of forehead then move them downward along the side of nose, move palms outward in small circles moving outward and upward from the chin then down to the chin beside the nose then upward on outside of face.

4. Massage eyes – First, run side of index finger along the bone above each eye. Second, pull tips of three middle fingers gently across eyes from the center toward outside edge. Third, pull side of index finger along ridge of bone below each eye. Rest thumbs on temples to support your hands during movement.

5. Massage ears from top to bottom by holding edge of ear between thumb and index finger. Pull top of ear upward then massage around outside edge of ear to stimulate pressure points for the whole body. Squeezing and releasing the ear lobe is good for headache and helps prostate or ovaries. Pulling upward on earlobe also helps vertebrae of neck and releases neck pain.

6. Stroke sides of nose - thumbs at top of nose, stroke along sides of nose until thumbs are at bottom edge of nose then stroke upward to starting point. Repeat 36 times. Be sure to stroke the whole length of the nose including the points at

bottom of nose where the sides flare out. Pinching from the ridge of nose along top of nose 36 times has the same effect.

7. Hands on top of ear opening with fingers pointing backward. Tap back of head just above occipital process by placing tip of middle finger on head, index finger atop middle finger then snapping index finger down to skull. Ming tian gu - pat drum of heaven.

8. Stroke area over liver starting from top, outside edge toward center palms on torso, fingers angled downward toward mid line at 45 degrees, stroke across liver 36 times.

9. Stroke area over liver starting from top, outside edge toward center.

10. Stroke area over kidneys by making a fist then using the thumb and index finger side of fist to massage kidneys with up and down movements.

11. Circles hands on abdomen. First slowly and softly circle hands to right 50 times with circles getting smaller and smaller (builds yang) then either 25 or 50 circles to left (builds yin). Doing lying down is best either upon waking in the morning or just before sleep at night.

12. Run fingertips through hair from forehead to neck. At end of third stroke move hands away as if throwing off water to throw bad qi away.

13. Tap back of head just above occipital process by placing tip of middle finger on head, index finger atop middle finger

then snapping index finger down to brain. Thirty-six taps is best. This movement increases wisdom, wakes up spirituality.

14. Stroke area over liver starting from top, outside edge toward center.

15. Stroke area over kidneys by making a fist then using the thumb and index finger side of fist to massage kidneys with up and down movements.

16. Rub palm (Le gong) across sole of foot (yung chuan) – left hand across sole of right foot, right hand across sole of left foot. Back and forth from middle edge to outside and back.

17. Pat along your arms and legs - To accumulate qi pat up the outside of your arm with palm down (yang side) then down the inside (yin side) with Palm up. Repeat on the other arm. Pat down the outside of each leg from hip to knee. To release bad energy do the opposite on both arms and legs.

11 SMALL CIRCULATION OF HEAVEN QIGONG / XIAO ZHOU TIAN

Small Circuit of Heaven Qigong/*Xiao Zhou Tian* is a traditional Daoist qigong that has been practiced for centuries. The purpose of this qigong is to increase qi circulation. Small Circuit of Heaven qigong has the potential to open the Eye of Heaven (sometimes known to Americans as the third eye). This practice (*gong*) is advanced, therefore, it is recommended that only students who have practiced Happy Heart Qigong (*le xin gong*) seriously and daily attempt it. Knowledge of the process is not enough. Patience and unhurried practice over a long period of time is required to learn this extremely difficult gong. True understanding requires heart-to-heart transmission from teacher to student.

Position

Sitting on a cushion in lotus position is best. Women place right leg atop left and men place left leg atop right. Sitting cross-legged on a pillow is satisfactory. Sitting in a chair with legs bent to a ninety-degree angle, toes pointed straight ahead and legs open is also satisfactory. Erect posture is very important in Small Circuit of Heaven Qigong Small Circuit of Heaven Qigong although this is not important during Happy Heart Qigiong/ *le xin gong*.

When learning this gong hands can be held slightly above lap with palms facing upward and pad of thumbs touching. Women place right hand above left and men left above right. Later, the back of hands can be rested on the knees with palms facing up and thumbs touching the ring finger at the spot where it joins the palm.

Part 1 – Adjust Body/Tiao Shen
Use the same technique as in Happy Heart Qigong/ *le xin gong*.

Part 2 – Click Teeth/Kou Chi
Click teeth together 36 times.

Part 3 - Red Dragon Tongue Stirs the Sea/Chi Long Jiao Hai

1. Tongue is rotated outside the teeth clockwise then counter clockwise. 18 times in each direction is satisfactory, but 36 times in each direction is best. When tongue is at lowest point of circle begin inhalation through when tongue is at highest point in rotation. Exhale during downward half of circle.

2. Mouth is closed and tongue is rotated inside the teeth clockwise then counter clockwise 18 or 36 times in each direction.

3. Swallow saliva at any time during external or internal circling of tongue. If there is a great deal of saliva it is advantageous to swallow it in three swallows.

Part 4 – Relaxed Breathing/ Shu Xi Fa

Relax the body using the same technique as in *le xin gong*. Count your breaths. Beginners use 10 inhale/exhale cycles breathing in the same way as *le xin gong*. Over time, add inhale/exhale cycles in units of ten until 360 cycles can be completed comfortably. Counting the breaths helps promote calmness, focuses your intention, and contributes to accumulating *yuan qi* in your dantian.

Part 5 – Not Named by Shifu Cheng

The purpose of this part is to accumulate qi in the *dantian* then circulate it up the *du mai* meridian in the back and over the top of the head then down to the *ren mai* and back to the *dantian*. Once qi has accumulated circulation of qi can be attempted. This is exceptionally difficult. Typical problems in this stage random thoughts, too much intention, and not enough intention. Aides for calming random thoughts are think of your navel, look at the tip of your nose, or rest your mind in one area such as the Eye of Heaven/*yin tang* between the eyebrows, *dan zhong*, *dantian*, or Bubbling Well/*yong chuan* at the center of the sole of the foot. Any of these aides should be done for a very short time. Each can be repeated one or two additional times if needed. Being calm and relaxed is crucial when learning the optimum amount of intention. Thinking of qi flowing as a current of electricity can be helpful.

1. First, inhale using abdominal breathing and think of good energy to the *dantian*. Pausing before beginning exhalation is important. Exhale using *dantian* breathing and think of the *dantian* becoming warm or picture a hot ball of energy in the *dantian* or think of nothing. There is no pause before beginning the next inhalation. The *dantian* can become quite hot during this part of the gong. Some people feel a feeling of electricity rather than heat and some sense a golden ball. Each of these sensations is an indication that qi has accumulated.

2. Use your intention to send qi to the *hui yin* which is located near the perineum. As you send this qi, inhale to your *dantian* and raise your eyebrows and simultaneously roll your eyeballs as if gazing upward.

3. Intend qi to rise to the *chang jian* then mingmen at the waist, then a pressure point called the *jia jī zhuang* which is a little above the waist at the spine. Briefly draw in the perineum and simultaneously move tongue so it touches the top of the mouth to create bridges between the *du mai* and *ren mai* meridians. when attempting this segment of circulation. This helps qi go through the meridians and their branches.

4. Imagine *qi* continuing to rise up the *du mai*, a major meridian that runs up the back, to the *feng fu* or *yü gen* which is at the hollow in the back of the skull.

5. Imagine qi continuing to the Neiwan Palance/*nei wan gong* then up to the *bai hui*.

6. Once qi reaches this point begin slowly exhaling and intend qi to move to your *yin tang* which is between your eyebrows then to the *ren zhong* then down to your *dantian*.

7. Ideally, one inhalation is make as you circulate qi from the *hui yin* to *bai hui*, but multiple inhalations can be made if necessary. If multiple breaths are needed, exhale briefly before each inhale. The breath should be so light that it would not move a feather.

Part 6 – Closing/Shou Gong

This part is similar to the closing of Happy Heart Qigong *le xin gong* although there are some important changes. Rather than pulling energy at the level of *dan zhong*, place palms on the *dantian* and circle them clockwise then counterclockwise 81 times each. Women place right hand inside left, men place left hand inside right. Circle the palms on the eyes, but omit the other motions done in *le xin gong*. The nose is rubbed using up and down movement with sides of thumb using area between first and second joint. In *le xin gong* contact between thumb and nose is only on the down stroke. The ears are massaged in a small circle 14 times with palms flat against them. Rather than up and down hand movements to massage the kidneys place the palms over the *mingmen* with one palm on top of other flat over *mingmen* and circle them 91 times. The direction of the circle does not matter. Kidneys are massaged 91 times with the sides of fists.

In addition to the typical le *xin gong* closing as modified above massage the feet. First, pull each toe back toward the body starting with the big toe and working to the small to. It does not matter which foot is massaged first and the number of times does not matter. Second, rub the (what part of hand? Across the (what area near where toes join foot?) several times. Finally, rub the palm across the sole of the foot 90 times for each foot with the Bubbling Well (*lao gong*) of the palm moving directly over the Bubbling Well (*yong quan*) of the sole of foot.

12 HAPPINESS QIGONG/LE GONG

This standing qigong set was developed by Shifu's qigong master, Master Kong Tai to promote movement of qi in the body. The Chinese character for *le* is the character that was on the t-shirts students wore in class for several years. *Le* is translated as happiness, joy, music, and peacefulness. Eventually the shirts were redesigned and *le* was replaced by a diagram of the bagua, the eight trigrams associated with the Eight Gates in tai chi chuan and which are components of the sixty-four hexagrams in *Yi Jing/I Ching*.

A heart-warming moment occurred on the day Shifu and Master Kong were reunited after a fourteen-year separation and just two months before her death. During his first public lecture in the USA Master Kong (speaking in Chinese to a Chinese audience) told the audience he'd had a special surprise earlier in the day when his long-lost disciple attended his press conference. He called Shifu to the stage. I did not understand what Master Kong said, but both of them wore enormous smiles. Shifu said something that I'm guessing was about the Center for Harmony t-shirts which she and the five students who accompanied her that day were wearing because she turned so everyone could see the large character for *le* (樂) on the back – the same character Master Kong which was a main theme in his lecture. The audience laughed. Shifu called her students to the stage to show off our shirts. Although I couldn't understand the words being said, it was easy to see the happiness and joy singing in Shifu's heart.

Preparation for Le Gong

1. Start with feet together, arms hanging loosely at your sides, hands relaxed and slightly cupped.

2. Gaze at the floor a few feet in front of you while keeping head straight. Keep your eyes open a little bit because you might fall down if they're closed. Focusing on a small spot helps you be calmer.

3. Tongue touching the top of your mouth.

4. Step to the left with left foot, right foot remains in place. By bending arms at the elbows, raise hands until your forearms are horizontal with palms facing down.

5. Move hands forward simultaneously circling each toward the outside and then back to starting position. Continue circling the palms. Imagine good energy from the earth entering through the palm (*lo gong*) then spreading through your arms and to the rest of your body.

6. After 5-10 cycles, reverse the direction.

First Form

1. Bring hands to rest at the dantian, palms facing inward. Women place left hand atop right and men place right hand on left.

2. Open hands outward in an arc by rotating your upper arms. Elbows stay near your side; however; arm pits are open to allow qi flow. At the end of the movement your palms face forward. (Think of this as the elbow being like the hinge of a door and the arm the door)

3. Retrace the same arc and return hands to the starting position at the dantian. Imagine bringing good energy to your dantian.

4. Inhale as you open your arms and exhale as they return to your dantian.

5. Repeat the opening and closing movements 5 to 10 times.

Second Form

1. From the ending position with hands on dantian, bring palms outward and move them upward in an arc until they reach the level of your heart.

2. Slowly separate the heels of your hands, with the middle fingers maintaining contact as the backs of the fingers roll together and your hands form fists touching at the backs of the fingers. The backs of the hands are now facing away from you.

3. Move the hands apart until the fists are at about shoulder width.

4. Open fists so that palms face each other with fingers pointing skyward then slowly bring palms toward each other until they are a few inches apart.
5. Make a fist in the same way as before and repeat, moving the fists apart.
6. Imagine good energy being expanded as your fists move apart and condensed as you palms move together. Think of bringing good energy to your heart area during these movements.
7. Repeat the opening and closing movements 5 to 10 times with palms coming together on the last closing motion.

Third Form

1. The closed palms from the previous form rise to the level of your eyebrows.
2. The motions of the second form are repeated. Imagine good energy for your brain to promote the development of wisdom.
3. Repeat the opening and closing movements 5 to 10 times with palms coming together on the last closing motion.

Fourth Form

1. Slowly drop the closed hands down the center line of your torso with palms gradually moving apart beginning with the heels of hands and ending with fingertips losing contact when hands are about the level of the waist.

2. Bring the hands slowly to your back and place the backs of your hands on the kidneys.

3. Raise the hand up the spine as high as they can go. When they can go no further, bring hands around in front and replace them behind your head/neck, again with middle fingers touching but now with palms facing your upper spine or neck. Continue moving the hands upward past the back of the head and over the top of the head.

4. As the hands pass your forehead, the palms face downward. Slowly lower them, palms down, in front of your body as the until they reach the dantian. Middle fingers point at each other; however, contact does not have to be maintained after the hands begin their downward movement.

5. Imagine the yin and yang energy of your body being balanced as your hands drop slowly down the mid line of your body.

6. Repeat the rising and falling movements of the hands 5 to 10 times. On the last downward movement the palms face downward at the level of the dantian.

Fifth Form

1. The downward facing palms from the ending of the previous form rotate upward and the arms extend forward until straight (but not locked). The arms are now horizontal with palms up.

2. Rotate the arms outward and bring the hands backward in a wide arc and place the palms on the kidneys.

3. Slide the palms down the back, over buttocks, down the back of legs to the knees, and around knees. Bend at the waist to allow palms to reach down legs.

4. Straighten the waist and slowly extend the hands forward as far as possible while simultaneously doing a deep knee bend. Go as far down as you can manage while keeping the back vertical.

5. As you slowly return to a standing position, again rotate the arms outward and bring the palms in a wise arc to the kidneys.

6. Repeat these movements 5 to 10 times.

Sixth Form

1. Bring palms together at the level of dantian with palms touching, one facing up and the other facing downward. Women have right hand below left and men have left hand below right. Close your eyes throughout this form.

2. Slowly separate the hands vertically until they are 8-12 inches apart, then bring them back towards each other to within an inch or two.

3. Imagine good energy for your heart during this form.

4. Repeat the expanding and contracting movements 5 to 10 times ending with both palms at level of dantian.

Seventh Form

1. From closing position for previous form, separate the hands slightly and rotate them to face the dantian. Hands do not touch the body.

2. Bring the hands up and away from the body in a gentle arc to the level of the eyes with your palms facing your eyes.

3. Keep the eyes open as you bring the palms to within an inch or two of the eyes while looking at the palm (lo gong).

4. Imagine good energy for the dantian when hands are near body and good energy for the eyes as the palms are being brought to the eyes.

5. Repeat these movements 5 to 10 times ending with palms near eyes.

Eighth Form

1. From the closing position of the previous form, move the hands to an inch or two above each kidney with palms facing the kidney. Think good energy for the kidneys.

2. Raise hands to an inch or two away from ears with palms facing the ears. Think good energy for the kidneys.

3. Repeat these movements 5 to 10 times ending with palms near the ears.

Ninth Form

1. From the closing position of the previous form, move hands to a few inches wider than the sides of and slightly in front of body with arms fully extended, palms down.

2. Rotate each hand with a scooping motion and lift hands to the nose thinking of a pleasant smell.

3. Repeat motion, however, lift hands to the mouth and think of good energy for the mouth.

4. Repeat motion, thinking of nothing.

Tenth Form

1. Fully extend and raise both arms into the air straight above the head.

2. Keep arms extended, but relaxed. Lower them to shoulder height WHILE simultaneously bending knees as far as possible for you. Keep the back straight and vertical throughout the motion. As you straighten the legs, return arms to starting position above your head.

3. Repeat these movements 5-10 times.

4. Think good energy for all the joints in your body.

Closing

1. Rotate the arms outward then raise extended, but relaxed arms from the sides to above the head and end with palms facing each other.

2. With middle fingers pointing at each other and palms facing downward, move hands slowly down the center line to the dantian.

3. Repeat this motion three times. During the first cycle think of balancing yin and yang energy. During the second cycle think of good energy for the internal organs of your body. During the third cycle think of good energy for your bei hui, yin tan, tan zhong, and dantian as your hands pass each of these areas.

4. Close with hands at dantian. Women have right hand on dantian with left hand atop right. Men have left hand on dantian and right hand atop left.

5. Press palms together at the heart with fingers pointing away from body and thinking closing.

6. Pat down the meridians of arms from shoulder to fingers then legs from thighs toward toes.

13 FIVE ELEMENTS QIGONG/ WU XING ZHANG

During a qigong workshop in China, Shifu was part of a small group selected to learn this qigong set from a master who brought these exercises from Wudan Mountain. She did not teach this set until a most students had been studying with her for several years because this is a highly secret, extremely powerful qigong. When she first started teaching this qigong Shifu cautioned students never to share these exercises with anyone outside Center for Harmony. Later, she included people who attended class only once with no apparent concern about keeping it secret. The entire set can be done any time of year. Also, it is fine to do 1, 2, 3, or 4 parts as long as they are done in the order of the seasons they represent.

Sounds

"Sound" is the vibration formed in the mouth by silently forming the sound. Pitch does not matter.

- Spring - Liver – *xu* (In English sounds like shoe or shuuuuuuuuu)
- Summer - Heart – *he* (In English sounds like huuuh)
- Long Summer - Spleen – *hu* (In English sounds like who)
- Autumn - Lung – *si* (In English sounds like saaaah) -
- Winter - Kidney – chui (In English sounds like chuei, think each sound . . . ch, short u, ah, long e))
- Sixth Sound - Sanjao – *xi* (say shheeeee) Shifu Cheng indicated there is no adequate translation for san jiao which is a single unit comprised of the upper, middle, and lower dantian. She said the typical translation of san jiao as Triple Burner is a mistranslation.

Preparation/Warm Up for Any Season

1. Purpose – makes more saliva, increases enzyme production
2. Procedure
   a. Teeth – chatter (36 times)
   b. Tongue
      i. Turn inside mouth - 9 to left then to 9 right
      ii. Turn outside mouth - 9 to left then to 9 right
      iii. Do total of 4 sets of 9 left/9 right, inside and outside

c. Swallow saliva three times, send to *dantian*

d. Hair – comb fingers through it in same manner as at end of qigong (36 times)

e. Palms –

    i. rub together then rub face in same manner as at end of qigong (36 times)

    ii. Start at chin, up outside of face, down center

Spring – Clear Liver

1. Feet shoulder width apart

2. Hands together at *dantian*, palms up with middle fingers touching

3. Shift weight to right foot, turn toward left corner

4. Step left/heel touch left foot

5. Push hands toward corner while shifting weight to left foot and silently forming the sound shuuuu (breathing out). Mouth is rounded at beginning of shuuu and broadens into almost a smile at the end of this silent sound.

6. When pushing hands (palms standing) away open eyes wide and imagine bad energy exiting through palm lo gung.

7. Once hands are fully extended transfer weight back to right foot and bring left foot back to shoulder width. Imagine good energy entering a simplified notion of the liver meridian – in big toe, up inside of leg, splitting into two streams near *dantian* and going up sides of torso to level of liver. Do this while inhaling. Also, lift big toe of left foot while breathing in.

8. Shift weight to left foot and repeat the process above toward the right.

9. Do at least six repetitions (to left and to right = one repetition), but ten is better.

Summer – Clear Heart

1. Feet shoulder width apart.

2. Hands start on left side of body with palms standing and facing outward.

3. Move hands across front of body toward right side as you take one step to the right.

4. Exhale while silently saying "huuuh" as hands move across front of body and imagine bad energy exiting the body.

5. At end of crossing body movement, hands rotate to palms up position with middle fingers touching.

6. Hands move to left as left foot is brought to meet the right foot. Inhale as this motion is occurring and imagine good energy entering the body.

Long Summer – Clear Spleen

1. Feet shoulder width apart.

2. Right knee comes up as high as possible simultaneously with right hand being lifted and inhaling. Sharply inhale while this motion is being made.

3. Be sure to keep your shoulder down when hand is being lifted.

4. Step forward onto right foot as hand moves across body toward right with palm facing your face. Exhale while silently saying "hu" as this motion is being made.

5. Repeat steps 2, 3, and 4 stepping left and bringing left hand across body.

Autumn – Clear Lungs

1. Feet should width apart.

2. Extend left hand to front and right hand toward back, waist turns toward right.

3. Step forward onto left foot while bringing hands together so that right hand crosses above left. Area just behind wrist of right hand crosses over same area on left hand.

4. Silently say the sound "si" while making movement in step 3.

5. Fingers of both hands gradually pinch together while making this step and ar fully pinched at the time of wrists crossing.

6. Fingers begin unpinching as the right hand extends forward and left extends backward. Unpinching is completed at the moment of full extension. Inhalation occurs as this extension occurs.

7. Repeat these steps on the other side.

Winter – Clear Kidney

1. Always start to left
2. Hands at *dantian*, move hands to left - turning waist actually moves the arms/hands, silently breathing out "Chuei".
3. Palms facing down with fingers curving up yet relaxed, toes up.
4. Movement is done walking (10 steps daily)
5. Step left for first full circle.
6. Silently, breath out forming the sound chuei. The long e sound is the longest part of the sound and continues until the arms/hands have moved all the way to right. The arc of the exhaling phase is wide.
7. Once the exhale has been completed, inhale through nose with tongue touching top of mouth. The arms/hands move from right to left in a small arc close to body.
8. When hand returns to *dantian*, right foot comes to center, then step right as chuei movement starts to left.
9. Be sure to turn the waist as hands move from side to side.
10. Imagine good energy entering through the mingmen on the inhale and bad energy exiting the body through the palm lo gong on the exhale.

14 QIGONG SPECIFIC TO SEASON

QIGONG FOR SPRING

Lower Blood Pressure/Prevent High Blood Pressure

This qigong can promote healthy blood pressure, prevent or heal heart disease especially rapid heart beat. It is best done after qigong. If you don't have time for qigong rub your hands together until your palms are hot then do this qigong. Do this or the liver strengthening qigong – not both.

1. Rub palms together 64 times.
2. Hold left hand in front of dantian and right in front of middle dantian (*dan zhong*). Both about 10 cm/4 inches from body. Do not touch your body.
3. Briefly think of red color going to your heart.
4. Do this for 10 minutes.
5. Close by bringing palms together at *dan zhong* then dantian

Strengthen Liver (Lā Qi or Push Good Energy)

This qigong is primarily to clear the liver. It can also be done to lower blood pressure and to heal a feeling bloated from gas in the abdomen. It is best done immediately after Happy Heart Qigong (*le xin gong*) because you are already filled with energy. This is good to do at the start of spring, but do the blood pressure qigong below unless you feel bloated. Do this or the blood pressure qigong – not both.

1. Remaining seated after qigong or standing are equally acceptable when doing this qigong. If you stand your feet should be shoulder width apart and the little finger of each hand should be on your legs a little in front of the midline on the side of each leg.

2. Breathe naturally.

3. Slowly move your hands apart and together to a fewer inches apart with palms facing each other at roughly the level of the dantian. Do this until your hands become warm or you can sense energy between the *lo gong* in the center of your palms. Continuing without a sensation of qi between you lo gong is not as effective as waiting until you feel qi.

4. Bring your palms together then slowly move your left hand to your dantian and allow it to remain there. Simultaneously move your right hand so that it is eight to ten inches from your body with the palm facing your liver and hold your hand still and imagine it being the sun shining light toward your liver. Next, slowly move your hand toward then away from your liver for three to five minutes. Use your intention to pushing good energy to your liver when your hand moves toward your liver.

5. Close by placing both hands on the dantian then press palms together over danzhong/middle dantian.

QIGONG FOR SUMMER (<u>NOT</u> LONG SUMMER)

<u>Strengthen Heart</u>

This qigong is primarily to clear the heart. It is best done before Happy Heart Qigong/*le xin gong*. It should not be done before *xiao zhou tian*. It is best to do the heart strengthening qigong and *le xin gong* in the morning and *xiao zhou tian* in the evening. Heart strengthening qigong should be done daily during summer, but not in long summer.

1. Sit down facing south, close your eyes, relax your body.
2. Hands in the starting position for Happy Heart Qigong/*le xin gong*.
3. Click teeth together nine times.
4. Imagine red color filling your mouth then swallow saliva to the dantian. Do this three times.
5. Begin Happy Heart Qigong/*le xin gong* as normal.
6. Close by placing both hands on the dantian then press palms together over danzhong/middle dantian.

AUTUMN QIGONG

<u>Strengthen Lungs</u>

This qigong is done immediately upon waking up in the morning during the autumn. This is the most advantageous time because yang is low. Brush teeth before doing this qigong. Shower before doing this qigong if you plan to shower. This qigong can be done before Happy Heart Qigong/ *le xin gong* or *xiao zhou tian*. Caring for lungs in autumn will improve kidneys later. This qigong will also balance yin and yang in the whole body.

1. Sit with hands resting upon the knees, palms up with thumbs at the place where the ring finger joins the palm. It is acceptable to stand rather than sit.
2. Tongue touching top of mouth
3. Face west. If you are outside face trees. If inside, face outside if possible.
4. With eyes open, imagine seeing white light coming toward you. Simultaneously, place your middle fingers on the min tian quo (spot on back of head that is flicked in self-massage after qigong) and snap index fingers onto head from atop middle finger. Do this snapping motion seven times. When the light arrives close your eyes and begin to inhale the white light into your nose to your mouth. Once the mouth is filled with white light swallow saliva and imagine it carrying white light to your lungs then dantian. If you don't have enough

saliva it is okay to think of the white light flowing to the lungs on its own.

5. Exhale and silently think the sound "si" (like in wu xing/five elements qigong for lung). Hold saliva in your mouth during the exhale.

6. Slowly, complete seven cycles of inhale and exhale.

7. Think of dantian being warm

8. Close with palms together at *dan zhong* (middle dantian).

If you have time you can add any of the following:

1. Add tooth click (*ko chr*) 36 times

2. Add tongue circling like *xiao zhou tian*

3. Add breathing of 36 inhale/exhale cycles to *dan tian* like in *xiao zhou tian* without the white light. On exhale make the silent sound of "si"

4. Tap back of head 36 times in the manner done after le xin gong.

WINTER QIGONG

<u>Strengthen Kidneys</u> - Gu Shen Bu Xu Gong

1. Stand naturally and calmly with feet together then step to feet to shoulder width apart.

2. Hands start at sides, raise to level of *dan zhong* where palms come together. Rub palms together 36 or more times.

3. Breathe naturally

4. Place palms on the kidney – mingmen area and hold them there for several seconds (30-60) then rub the area by moving hands up and down thirty-six times slowly. Use more pressure and intent on the down stroke than on the up stroke.

5. Turn hands with the back of the hand on the kidneys with hands relaxed and fingers curled slightly but not touching.

6. Hold this position for at least 20 minutes with a eyes gazing at the floor a bit in front of you or a eyes closed. Closed is best.

7. Think of qi being stored in the kidney, jing being stored in the kidney, kidney qi being cleared.

8. To end, bring hands to *dan zhong* with palms together, hands go to dantian with palms on dantian.

9. Turn hands facing upward with middle finger nearly touching. Raise hands to level of *dan zhong*, turn them down and return to *dantian*. Do this three times.

10. Palms on dantian to close.

QIGONG FOR ANY SEASON

Strengthen Stomach

This qigong is good if you have stomach problems. It is best done an hour after a meal.

1. Start with fee shoulder width apart.

2. Palms face abdomen about 5 inches/10 cm away and 3 to 3.5 inches apart
   a. Women have right hand inside of left
   b. Men have left hand inside of right
3. All toes except big toes grip the floor.
   a. Women grip with right foot first then left
   b. Men grip with left foot first then right
4. Hold this position for 10 minutes.
5. Close by bringing your palms to the dan tian.
   a. Women place right hand under left
   b. Men place left hand under right

Strengthen San Jiao

This qigong clears your *san jiao* and promotes energy flow to all five zang organs (liver, heart, spleen, lungs, kidney). The best time to do this qigong is between 9:00 – 11:00 pm when cosmic energy is coming to the *san jiao*, however, it is beneficial for your body any time of the day.

1. Stand naturally with feet together and relax your whole body.
2. Step left to shoulder width apart.
3. Bring hands together in front of pubic bone or a bit higher with middle fingers touching, palms up and forming sort of an imaginary basket.

4. Raise hands to the level of *dan zhong* and rotate on the axis of middle fingers and push hands over your head until your arms are fully extended.

5. Exhale and silently say xi (prounced sheeeee) from the start up the upward movement until it completes.

6. Once highest point is reached, bring arms to the side while slowly inhaling.

7. Inhale through the time you are lowering your arms.

8. Imagine good energy entering body through the meridians that start in the two outside toes on both feet when exhaling. Toes grip the earth.

9. Perform these movements for at least six cycles.

15 MISCELLANEOUS TYPES OF QIGONG

PATTING QIGONG - TIAO SHEN GONG

The movements of this qigong are simple yet they have a strong effect on the body. It is an ancient Daoist qigong being popularized on television throughout China, Japan, and other countries by a Chinese man who journeyed in China to find masters to teach him traditional techniques after he became disillusioned by his work in the business world of New York City.

This gong can heal because it impacts the meridians. They are like the roots of a tree that cannot be seen. Pressure points cannot be seen either. If a person feels pain it means there is a block or stagnation in a meridian. There are twelve major meridians. *Jin* are horizontal meridians and *lou* are vertical meridians that are comparable to the rings of a tree. There is a close relationship between meridians and *zang fu*. *Du mai*, *ren mai*, and three major meridians   down   the   back   are   important.

When you pat yourself think of good qi going in and when you remove your hand think of bad qi going out. Think this for a short time. Pat must be hard enough to cause healing. When you pat yourself patting can cause the patted area to become red if stagnation is being released and even black if a lot is being released. Nourish the body with qi from food and air breathed in during qigong. Qi and *xue*/blood for bēn. All three are fundamental in the body. Qigong is good to make up qi in blood and good for circulation. Necessities for good health are good circulation in meridians, having qi in wuzang, and having qi in blood.

The order of patting is:

1. Top of head/*bai hui*
2. Sides of head
3. Back of neck
4. Each shoulder
5. Middle up upper arm on outer side, one arm at a time
6. Inside of arm just below line for elbow on left arm only (for heart)
7. Chest above breast (pat lightly)
8. Hips with arms hanging down and fully extended
9. Sides of each knee with two hands on one knee at a time
10. On the knee cap, one hand on each knee simultaneously (can be done sitting or standing bent)
11. Behind knee cap, one hand on each knee simultaneously (can be done sitting or standing bent)

STANDING QIGONG

Shifu taught this qigong to a small group of students who happened to be present early in the morning at a weekend-long retreat. She did not say the name or purpose of this qigong.

1. Stand with feet shoulder width, slightly bent, arms in front in circle

2. First – imagine qi moving around LEFT foot – start at little toe, back to heel where pause, continue to big toe then extend Yung chuan into earth to connect to Yin

3. Second – imagine qi circling head from left side of face at edge of scalp then around back to front starting point. Imagine reaching up like an antenna to connect to sun during day or moon at night.

4. Third – after connecting, imagine receiving Yang from sky, Yin from earth.

5. Fourth – imagine Yin/Yang energy circulating to internal organs, to blood, to body fluids, to cells

6. Fifth – imagine body getting larger and larger until it is One with Universe

7. Sixth – to close sink everything to *dantian*, press palms together, think closing.

8. Can also be done during le gong

9. Best done at least 20 minutes

10. If done regularly, lots of good energy will result, etch individual must pay attention to her own experience. Teacher can teach the process, but student must find out what it means

11. Once the connection is made calmly relax your entire body and allow it to expand into oneness with the universe.

QIGONG FOR PREVENTING OR HEALING STROKE

Two qigong techniques can prevent stroke or help with healing after a stroke occurs. These techniques are supplemental techniques that can be added when doing sitting qigong.

Technique #1

1. Sitting position with hands resting on thighs, palms up. Sitting on the floor is best, however, it can be done in a chair especially if you are sick.

2. While doing qigong be aware of *qi*/feel *qi*

3. The sound *weng* (pronounced wung in English) accompanies this process. The sound is made silently in the same manner as the sounds in Five Elements/*wu xing*. Inhale when breath runs out and continue the silent sound.

4. Open the bei hui then allow qi to enter through the *bei hui*. This is the area in the top of the skull where your middle fingers touch if you put your thumbs at the highest point on your ears and spread your hand upward.

5. Once the qi is entering the *bei hui* think of it moving to *ren zhong* and changing to a white light

6. Intend the white light to go to the *ni wan*, the empty place in the brain a few inches below the *bei hui*, and then to the *tan zhong*.

7. Once the white light has reached the *tan zhong* imagine it changing to red light that spreads throughout your whole body.

8. Do this technique for ten minutes after *le xin gong* or *xiao zhou tian*.

Technique #2

1. Do this technique for ten minutes after *le xin gong* or *xiao zhou tian*.

2. The sound *ah* accompanies this process. The sound is vocalized softly with only the sound air leaving the body makes during exhaling.

3. Bring qi in through *bei hui* then imagine it splitting into two streams.

4. Each stream goes down each leg to top of foot then out *lo quan* on sole of foot.

Technique #3

1. While doing qigong be aware of *qi*/feel *qi* and think of it entering the *bei hui*.

2. The sound *xu* (pronounced shoe in English) accompanies this process. The sound is made silently in the same manner as the sounds in Five Elements/*wu xing*

3. The eyes are open as if you are angry.

4. Inhale *qi* to the *lin tan* while turning the head to the left.

5. Exhale while returning head to center/facing forward and silently saying xu.

6. Inhale while turning head to right.

7. Exhale while returning head to center/facing forward and silently saying xu.

8. Think of qi going to your big toe when turning to the left and long chuan when turning to the right.

9. Do this technique for five minutes after *le xin gong* or *xiao zhou tian*.

10. This technique helps circulation in the brain and blood vessels.

ARM SWINGING QIGONG

Shifu did not tell students the name of the qigong or what it is for, but she indicated it is powerful in spite of its simplicity.

1. Stand with arms at sides, sidestep.

2. Swing arms back then forward five times

3. On sixth swing forward and back, dip knees coordinated with swing back and again with swing forward.

4. Repeat several times.

In fall, this qigong can be combined with the fall qigong for lungs in which light is brought into the mouth.

1. 1st – autumn qigong facing west

2. 2nd – arm swing qigong

3. 3rd – swing arms to simultaneously hit dantian and mingmen 36 times. This is done with moving hands in an arc so that the hits are alternated between right and left hands.

CLEAR LIVER & GALL BLADDER MERIDIAN

Shifu introduced this qigong in spring with no explanation except that it clears the liver

1. Start with feet together then step with left foot to have feet at shoulder width.

2. Close eyes

3. Position One

   a. Slowly, slowly make small circles with hands starting at dantien, palms down, right hand moves clockwise and left counterclockwise.

   b. Imagine palm *lo gung* and foot *yuan chuan* being together.

   c. Do this until you feel heat or energy moving for up to five minutes.

4. Position Two

   a. Feet remain in same position as Position One, still shoulder width

   b. Eyes closed

   c. Press palms together at middle dantian/*danzhong*

   d. Think "good energy" in your palms

5. Position Three

    a. Feet remain in same position as Position One, still shoulder width

    b. Eyes closed

    c. Hands a few inches in front of liver with palms facing torso, right hand below left with fingers of right hand pointing left and fingers of left hand pointing right.

    d. Inhale while imagining good energy moving from palm *lo gung* into liver, also imagine this energy being green.

    e. Exhale bad energy down the legs and out feet yuan chuan, send the bad energy deep into the earth

    f. Continue for about five minutes.

6. Position Four – to bring good energy to kidney

    a. Feet remain in same position as Position One, still shoulder width

    b. Eyes closed

    c. Hands on back with palms touching kidney area (just above waist), fingers pointing toward center

    d. Think good energy into kidney

    e. Can also massage the pressure point for kidney by touching pressure point (it will feel discomfort when the pressure point is pressed) moving finger in small circles on the pressure point.

7. End

    a. Palms press together at middle dantian

    b. Step together

16 QIGONG AND INTENTION/YI

Entering a calm state is the first goal of qigong. Intention/*yi* means focusing attention on one spot then briefly thinking something such as moving qi to the dantian or intending qi to flow to a part of your body that doesn't feel well if you are ill. Focusing intention too long or too intensely can interfere with relaxation which, in turn, interferes with taking in qi. The more relaxed you are the more qi you receive.

During qigong, intention is used gently to help channel qi where it is needed. Qigong intention is a physical state in which movement of qi is guided. Using intention is similar to prayer, but prayer is spiritual only.   Meditation also involves entering a calm state; however, it does not involve using intention.

Intention is used differently in different types of qigong. Some types use a little for a short time, some for a long time, some not at all. When doing qigong it is best to mix times of non-action/*wu wei* and *you wei*. *Wu wei* means being calm and relaxed and not using your intention. *You wei* means using your intention for a short time. When you use your intention avoid serious, intense focus since this works against the relaxation that is part of qigong. For example, if you think of a lotus in your abdomen filling with light simply think briefly about the lotus rather than strongly thinking over and over again the lotus is filling with light, the lotus is filling with light.

Calming your emotions supports your intention. Good thoughts and bad thoughts might arise during qigong. Two types of good, helpful thoughts might arise one is thinking of things outside your body such as our river, a flower, a mountain, or other things in nature. The other type of helpful thinking is noticing what is happening inside you. Bad or unhelpful thinking are emotions or thoughts about difficulties in daily life. If fear arises during qigong, stop the thought. If you think of a dead loved one stop the thought. Allowing thoughts such as these to continue brings bad energy. If you cannot stop your emotions or difficult thoughts you should stop doing qigong at that time.

17 CHINESE NATURAL HEALTH CULTURE

This chapter consists of transcriptions of class notes from the Chinese Natural Health Culture series that occurred at MacDuffie School from November 2009 through May 2010. Student Xia Tang assisted with translation during most of these lectures. Class notes presented in this chapter consists of class notes from those lectures. Transcriptions are as close as possible what Shifu taught during lectures.

LECTURE #1
DIFFERENCES BETWEEN CHINESE AND WESTERN MEDICINE

Understanding differences between Chinese and western medicine is important for people who play taijiquan or practice qigong meditation because both are components of traditional Chinese medicine. Although the Cultural Revolution was a time of enormous difficulty for me, I was lucky too because the difficulties actually created the opportunity for me to study books about both Chinese and western medicine.

My first husband's parents were skilled physicians trained in western medicine in Japan. The Communists forced them to denounce each other. They were each angry with the other for the bad things they were forced to say and they separated. Their personal medical library was given to my husband. There was a period when I was extremely ill and too sick to work. I spent this time studying the medical library that was in my home and learned about western medicine.

In 1977, after the Cultural Revolution ended the government assigned me the job of assembling a public library. I was given an amount of money each month with which to purchase books. I bought many types of books. I bought books I thought others would like and books I wanted to read. Many people thought this was not a good job, but I was very lucky because I was often able to study all day long.

I read books about traditional Chinese philosophy such as the *Five Classics (Wu Jing)*, *Daode Jing* by Lao Tzu and the *Four Books (Si Shu)* of Confucian philosophy which included *The Great Learning/Da Xue* and

The Doctrine of the Mean/ Zhong Yong. These books had information about how a good person lives and the importance of being calm and emotionally well balanced.

I also read books about the traditional Chinese health culture and, to me, these were the best. For example, I read *Yi Jing/I Ching* which is a philosophy of nature – a combination of natural and social science that encompasses everything. I learned about five elements, eight directions, and bagua. Bagua (triagrams) are made of broken lines that represent yin and solid lines that represent yang. I also learned that each person is a small universe and that both the large universe and each person have energies called jing, qi, and shen. It took a long time to understand and a great deal of study because I had no teacher.

My interest in traditional Chinese medicine began when I was a child. My uncle was a doctor of Chinese medicine. Also, I accompanied my father when he visited a neighbor who had a Chinese medicine shop. While my father talked with his friend I explored the shop for interesting things. In those days Chinese doctors went to people's homes so they could see the family members and the home environment because it gave clues to understanding the illness.

Currently in China, traditional medicine is less important than western medicine. In 1950, Mao Zedong elevated western medicine over traditional Chinese medicine. By 1958, medical universities were established that favored using western-style machines to diagnose problems over traditional methods. Western medicine diagnoses and treats the site of a health problem. The body is treated like a machine that has parts that can be repaired. For example, chemotherapy is used to treat cancer, however, this kills healthy cells along with cancer cells. Traditional Chinese medicine favors a holistic approach that uses pulses, tongue color, frequency and consistency of bowel movements, urine, color of the skin, and possibly the *feng shui* of a person's physical environment to diagnose problems that western machines cannot identify. Considering interrelationships within the whole body is important. For example, fire in the heart due to excessive anger eventually causes a health problem. Healing the liver is necessary to address the problem with the heart.

Last year when I was in China I was sick, probably because of the bad air. I was unable to do qigong because of the prevalence of cigarette smoke. A friend told me to go to a western hospital, but I refused. In western medicine, patients submit to the physician. I was afraid they would keep me and give me lots of western medicine and I would die there. Instead, I went to a Buddhist doctor then went home to heal myself.

As mentioned earlier, western medicine is a major subject in Chinese universities and instruction about traditional medicine is weak.

Western medical students learn by dissecting cadavers, often of people who were sick. Chinese medicine is best learned through experience. Some masters can actually see the colors of internal organs inside a living body. Learning philosophy, spirituality, and about the outside culture are all required. Chinese medicine is grounded in understanding the mysteries within the body as well as natural law. Learning Dao is important. There are many paths within the philosophy of Dao. The Dao in which you heal yourself is one path. This path requires that you understand yourself so you can heal yourself by adjusting your emotions, food intake, and sleep patterns. Routines of your daily life such as doing qigong, playing taiji, and wearing clothes that keep your body warm are important parts of this path.

The *Yi Jing/I Ching* says that change in humans is constant because changes in nature are constant. Learning to be calm, relaxed, and balanced helps you deal with changes. Traditional Chinese medicine promotes wholeness and harmony within the body and within the universe.

LECTURE #2
UNDERSTANDING YOURSELF

The first task for my students is to understand yourself on the outside and inside. If you believe you might get sick and believe doctors and hospitals will cure you then you are more prone to health problems. If you understand yourself on the inside and outside you can promote your own normal health by helping your body have its own rhythm. By looking inside yourself you can understand yourself physically (internal organs) as well as mentally (personal characteristics such as emotions). If you understand yourself and your health then you can understand everything. Some people are very smart and have a lot of knowledge, but do not understand themselves. Without understanding yourself and how to keep healthy you can become ill and you may die.

The traditional Chinese health culture provides a way of understanding yourself. The principles are described in ancient books such as the *Huang Di Neijing* (Yellow Emperor's Internal Classic) and the *Yi Jing/I Ching* (Book of Changes). I have studied these important and essential books and am teaching my students about the treasures of this health culture.

Today, few people understand the principles in these books even in China. I observed an example of not understanding yesterday when I was riding on the highway in Connecticut. It was unseasonably warm day and I saw a man driving his convertible with the top down. This man did not understand the relationship between cold and illness because western medicine does not consider these principles. The man did not understand that cold, windy conditions are not good for health because they allow the meridians and pressure points to become cold.

The western view is that the human body is like a machine and doctors perform operations to perform broken parts. Western physicians do tests to diagnose the symptoms then prescribe medicine that does nothing to change the person energetically. The view of traditional Chinese medicine is that a person is a person and not a machine. In each person the blood, energy, and organs function in relationship to each other. Each person is different and each needs to change in a way that corresponds to her or his personal health needs. Later I will talk about these in detail.

During Small Circle of Heaven Qigong/*xiao zhoutian* I have been teaching how to circulate qi within two major meridians. The *du mai* which goes up the back is particularly important for men. The *ren mai* which goes down the front is particularly important for women. When western doctors deliver a baby via Cesarean section the *ren mai* and some other meridians are cut and this is very serious. The *du mai* and *ren mai* come together at a pressure point called the *ren zhong*. This point is a little bit inside your face behind the area just under your nose. This pressure point is very important in Chinese medicine. In fact, situations have been recorded when a person has died and been brought back to life by a physician who knows the technique of pinching the area in front of the *ren zhong*. There are methods to change the *ren zhong* in ways that increase the length of life and promote quality of health such as clearing the body, exercise, and eating well.

There are many types of Chinese doctors. Some heal the mind, some the body, and some both. Those who treat both are considered to be the highest doctors. Studying the *Dao De Jing/Tao Te Ching* can teach about the internal workings of the body. Sigmund Freud said you have to understand yourself. Understanding yourself was part of Chinese culture for thousands of years before Freud. Some people think learning about yourself internally is boring, but it is important knowledge. I hope my students are serious about learning Chinese health culture because taiji and qigong are important parts of this culture.

LECTURE #3
BEING & NON-BEING

There are two fundamental categories of the universe - non-being (*wu*) and being (*you*). These can also be understood as nothingness and substance. Ancient people determined these categories using physical eyes and the eye of heaven (*tian yian*) located between the eyebrows. Physical eyes can see only one-third of the universe. Something not physical can be seen only by using the eye of heaven to see or to know internally (*nei zhen*).

Practicing qigong can open the eye of heaven. Seeing with this eye is a natural ability when humans are born, but vision from this eye becomes obscured after birth. Scientific methods have proven what ancient people discovered. Modern equipment can measure what ancients could see with the eye of heaven.

The ancients understood that there is a relationship between the life of the universe and the life of a human being and that the human body is a small universe that functions in ways that parallel the universe. Lao Tze's *Daode Jing* describes this philosophy.

Internal Proof

Internal proof /*nei zheng*, or internal confirmation, is the basis of traditional Chinese medicine. Internal proof seen with the eye of heaven was used to understand the internal structure of the human body. Ancients using internal proof could see the energy flow among internal organs. They observed humans and determined how disease begins and how to cure it. Internal proof was extended via external proof by observing symptoms. They gradually developed the knowledge that disease can be cured by changing emotions which, in turn, changes and heals the physical body. Western medicine relies on cutting the body to relieve symptoms.

Fu Xi originated internal proof 8,000 years ago. He is credited with originating the eight trigrams that are the basis for the *Yi Jing/I Ching*. Very few people currently have the ability to use their eye of heaven to see internal proof. There are many stories about this. Ancients who had the ability gained fame because they cured people.

Qigong is a door to developing the ability to see internally with the eye of heaven. The eye will open only in people with a good heart. Those with an open eye of heaven can see energy coming from the stars as well as variations in energy flow at different times of the day. Within the human body can see energy moving in meridians, energetic connections among the internal organs, and variations of energy flow to internal organs at different times of the day.

Later, I will talk about what gives a person good energy. For now, it is important for my students to understand the relationship between their bodies and the universe. As humans develop more and more desire it pulls them away from the original nature that included ability to use the eye of heaven. Every religion has people who can see internally with the eye of heaven. In China, it was Taoists and Buddhists who developed this ability. The first goal of doing qigong is to heal yourself. Over a long period of time you may develop internal vision.

Present Life

There are three major parts of a human. The first is your original spirit (*yuan shen*) that you received from the universe and which will always continue with the universe. The second is your natural self. This is the yin and yang and five elements that you received from the natural universe. The third is the physical body that you received from your father and mother.

Internal vision can be used to heal spirit (*shen*). Western medicine only heals the physical body. 6,400 years ago pictures were developed that show the relationship between the Milky Way and the *mingmen* which is the major door to the human body. I will talk about this later.

LECTURE #4
WHAT ANCIENT PEOPLE SAW WITH
THE EYE OF HEAVEN

Human Body as a Small Universe

About 8,000 years ago, ancient Chinese philosophers developed the concept of the human body as a small universe that parallels the universe. Written characters or radicals were developed that depicts key relationships. Three words are important *tian* which means heaven

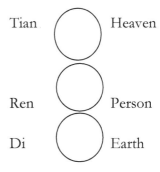

Tian — Heaven

Ren — Person

Di — Earth

or sky, *ren* which means person, and *di* which means earth. All three are joined when a person does qigong or plays tai chi. The Chinese characters for these words are intended to show the close relationship between humans and heaven.

The Energy of the Heavens

Each of the many stars in the heavens emits energy. In ancient times, many people had the ability to see this energy (*nei zhong*) including the color of the energy. Right now, there are a few people who can see the energy emitted by stars. People using the Eye of Heaven can see *tai yang xue* – beams of light the size of mung beans go directly from the sun or other stars to the temples on the side of each person's head. Energy also goes up the back, over the head and down to the heart.

People with inner vision (*nei zhong*) use the Eye of Heaven to see inside the human body and can see energy circulating among the five internal organs. Observing this flow of energy enables them to understand the energetic relationship of the organs. Traditional Chinese medicine is intended to support this relationship and strengthen the flow of energy that promotes human health. On the other hand, Western medicine is intended to kill pathogens and the unintended result is that healthy cells are also killed.

LECTURE #5
HUMANS AND THE MILKY WAY

There is a close relationship between humans and the Milky Way because good energy is sent from it to humans every day. This energy is sent to the *mingmen*. *Ming* translates to English as life and men means door. Energy sent daily to the door of life is important. The reality of this relationship is known via internal proof (*nei zhong*) through which people can see with their Eye of Heaven (*tian yian*).

Doing qigong calmly increases the chance that your eye of heaven will open.

Ancients could see three low walls (*san heng*) that are made of constellations. These walls are related to one another, however, each is in its own space. The first wall (*tian wei heng*) is like the central government. It is has twenty constellations made from seventy-eight major stars and twelve minor stars for a total of one hundred stars. (*xin zoa*). The second wall (*tian shi heng*) can be thought of as a market. It is has nineteen constellations made from eighty-seven major stars and one hundred and seventy-three minor stars. The third wall (*zi wei heng*) is very important. It can be thought of as a palace.

The North Star (Polaris) is the center of the sky. Around it are four sets of seven constellations. Each set of constellations has a different number of stars. The north has thirty-five major stars, the east has thirty-two, south had sixty-four, and west has fifty-one. Each set of constellations also has many minor stars.

The constellations and stars that make up the Three Walls are important because they control the heavens and they send energy to each person. The energy is sent in small balls the size of mung beans. The five stars named below plus the sun and moon all send energy to each human body and are considered to be the governors of the body.

The sun is the center of the sky. Human eyes can see the intense yellow light that is sent to each human every day from the sun. Some people can use their eye of heaven to see that in this energy from the sun is *taiyang* energy that enters the body through the temples.

Taiyang gives original energy, five elements energy, and yang energy to meridians – the gall bladder and intestine meridians, in particular. *Taiyang* moves through the up the back and along the back of the arms through the bladder meridian which is also called the sun meridian. *Taiyin* energy comes from the moon to the spleen and kidney meridians. The moon has a close relationship with women and menstruation.

In addition to energy from the sun and moon, humans receive energy from five major stars. The wood star sends green energy to the liver, fire star sends orangish red energy to the heart, earth star sends yellow energy to the spleen, metal star sends white energy to the lungs, and the water star sends black energy to the kidneys.

LECTURE #6
CONSTELLATIONS AND HUMAN BODY

In ancient China people identified four groups of seven constellations. Each group of seven constellations can be thought of as a house with a family in each. Each constellation can be thought of as a dormitory in the body. Each of group has a shape that organizes the constellations for that direction. In the east a green dragon organizes constellations that are busy in spring. In the south a red bird organizes constellations that are busy in summer. In the west a white tiger organizes constellations that are busy in fall. In the north a black turtle organizes constellations that are busy in winter.

Each cardinal direction has a set of seven constellations. The Black Tortoise constellations in the north are Dipper/Dou, Ox/Niú, Maiden/Nu, Void/Xū, Rooftop/Wēi, Encampment/Shì, and Wall/ Bi. The White Tiger constellations in the west are Legs/Kuí, Bond/Lóu, Stomach/Wèi, Rooster's Crown/Mǎo, Net/Bì, Turtle Beak/Zī, and Three Stars/Shēn . The Red Bird constellations in the south are Well/Jǐng, Ghost/ Guǐ, Willow/Liǔ, Star/Xīng, Extended Net/Zhāng, Wings/Yì, and Chariot/Zhěn. The Green Dragon constellations in the east are Horn/Jiǎo, Neck/Kàng , Root/Dǐ, Room/Fáng, Heart/Xīn, Tail/Wěi , and Winnowing Basket/Jī.

Each of the four sets of seven constellations is busy at a different time of the year. The eastern set is busy in the spring, southern set in the summer, western set in the fall, and northern set in the winter. Each set has a characteristic color. Each sends strong light and energy to humans at the time it is busy. Some ancients could see the fluctuation of energy throughout the year and drew diagrams of it.

Each set of constellations sends energy primarily to one of the five main internal organs of the human body. The northern set sends strong yin and yang to the kidneys and mingmen in the winter. You need to clear your kidneys and *mingmen* in the winter to make it easier for your body to receive the energy being sent to it. The eastern set sends energy to the liver in the spring. The southern set sends energy to the heart in the summer and to the spleen in the long summer period at the end of summer. The western set sends energy to the lungs in the spring. Spleen energy is also sent during the eighteen days at the start of each season.

These four sets of constellations move as a whole in a counterclockwise direction in the sky. Each set is very strong in the season in which it is busy. Although one set of constellations is busiest in each season, the others do not stop emitting energy and light so all have some energy movement throughout the year. *Feng shui* is based on the movement of these sets of constellations. Your birth time, date, and place result in energy that is specific to you. *Feng shui* can be used to determine the proper direction of the door of your home so that you get the proper energy based on the configuration at the time of your birth.

LECTURE #7
TIMES OF THE DAY

Understanding yin and yang as well at the five elements (*wu xin*) is very important. The body exchanges yin and yang and the five elements. Only people who practice qigong can truly understand yin and yang. These are true substances rather than philosophical words. Yin and yang are clear in the state of Being. Non-Being also has yin and yang which is known by internal proofs (*nei zheng*).

There are different kinds of ying and yang. There are three types of yin qi (*san yin*) and three types of yang qi (*san yang*). *Tai yang* is the strongest, *yang* has medium strength, and *shou yang* is the weakest. Similarly, *Tai yin* is the strongest, *yin* has medium strength, and *shou yin* is the weakest. Each type of yin and each type of yang has a different color.

Right now in western hospitals, genes are being studies. Genes have atoms that are 10^{-7} in size. Right now, people who have an open Eye of Heaven can use internal proof to see that there are small balls of yin or yang which change in an orderly way. These balls are above the size of mung beans. Yang balls move upward and yin move downward. These balls have a lot of movement so pictures of them cannot be drawn.

Your body is like a river that is very close to san ying and san yang. Your body has twelve major meridians that are like rivers. The meridians have six categories that correspond to the types of yin and yang qi. Tai yang is strong yang, yang ming is medium yang, and shou yang is weak yang. Tai yinis strong yand, yin ming is medium yin, and shou yin is weak yin. The outer side of the legs and arms have yang meridians and the inner side has yin meridians.

About 8,000 years ago yin and yang and the bagua were explained in the *I Ching*. *The Classic of the Yellow Emperor* (*Huang di Nei Jing*) explained the correspondence between the stars and internal organs. Wu xin (five elements). Internal proof showed what time of day is best for each type of energy to go to the internal organs of the human body. This became known by people who have an open Eye of Heaven who watched the colors of energy. The wood star gives energy that cultivates and refreshes the liver between 1:00-3:00. 11:00 am – 1:00 pm is the time when the heart is cultivated and refreshed. The heart controls the other organs. The liver and heart are two organs that need rest during the time of receiving energy. Other organs do not need to rest during the time of receiving energy such as 2:00 – 4:00 for small intestine, 3:00 – 5:00 for gall bladder, 7:00-9:00 for stomach, 9:00- 11:00 for spleen

LECTURE #8
TAIJI ORGANS

As explained previously, the human body is a small universe that parallels the natural universe. Both contain Being which can be seen, and Non-Being that which cannot be seen. The human body contains taiji organs that cannot be seen and are classified as Non-being. Major taiji organs are the three tan tiens – upper (lin tang), middle (dan zhong), and lower (dan tian). There are five secondary organs – a hidden blood pressure organ, palm bubbling well, foot bubbling well, and bei hui in top of head.

Taiji organs are spheres that are like the taiji symbol (taiji tu). Taiji organs function to receive energy then release it. These organs also organize and regulate energy so that life can continue. If there is a problem in these organs illness can develop.

In a previous lecture I explained that Fu Xi who lived 8,000 years ago used his eye of heaven (*tian yian*) to see internal proof of energy coming to earth from celestial bodies. Internal proof is used to gather information about the taiji organs. They are always round. Sometimes they are like light and sometimes they are like qi. Some are quite small while others are big. Taiji organs are constantly turning and stoppage occurs only if there is a problem in the body. I will mention now that the five elements (wu xing) are dynamic and always moving. Translation of the concept of movement from Chinese to English is difficult because the English word element represents something that is stagnant or motionless, however, it is the closest translation for the Chinese word *xing*. I will talk more about five elements in a future lecture.

People with internal proof can see that medicines used in traditional Chinese medicines travel through meridians to where healing is needed. Each medicine used in traditional Chinese medicine treats a specific pulse in the body and medicines are selected because internal proof has been used to identify the home to which they are drawn. For example, lemon is drawn to the gall bladder and spleen so it can be used to heal those organs. Chinese medicines are designed to help the body release bad energy. Taijii organs can become medicine for up to two days and assist in the process of rebalancing yin and yang and releasing bad energy. When a person performs the entire Yang Style 118 long form in taijichuan, taiji organs throughout the body are impacted in a beneficial way. This happens automatically with no thought or effort on the part of the taiji player.

Western medicine is quite different from traditional Chinese medicine. Western medicines are either all yang or all yin and they treat one specific symptom. Chinese medicine always combines medicines so that both yin and yang are impacted in a way that causes balance to be restored to whatever is causing a health problem.

Chang San Feng who developed taijiquan, practiced qigong. He used traditional Chinese healing methods and lived to be 400 years old. He was not famous because those who know Truth keep quiet and remain unseen.

18 NATURAL MEDICINE HEALTH CULTURE

This chapter provides transcriptions of the Natural Medicine Health Culture lectures that occurred at Church of Good Shepherd from June through December in 2011. Student Xia Tang assisted with translation during most of these lectures. Class notes presented in this chapter consists of class notes from those lectures. Transcriptions are as close as possible what Shifu taught during lectures.

LECTURE #1
UNDERSTANDING YOURSELF

It is important for serious qigong students to understand the Chinese theory that is the foundation for qigong. The components of this theory are understanding yourself, life, the universe, and qigong. There are no textbooks on this topic. I have a lifetime of experience that I want to share. You can go to a school to learn external information and about western medicine, but schools do not teach how to understand your living self. Traditional Chinese medical theory is different from western medicine. Traditional Chinese medicine is based on *The Yellow Emperor's Classic of Internal Medicine/huáng dì nèi jīng*. This tradition requires that you learn about yourself and philosophy.

In addition to the internal organs there are six aspects that define the difference between life and death. These are shén or spirit, jing or essence, qi or energy, xue or blood, jīn yè or bodily fluids, and jīn luò or a net of channels that transfer energy. If you do not have any one of the six aspects you will be dead. The body is like the universe. 2/3 cannot be seen in the universe and 2/3 cannot be seen in the body. Only xue/blood and jinye/bodily fluids can be seen, therefore, two-thirds of the aspects that define life cannot be seen.

1. Spirit/ shén is the governor of life. It includes intention, emotions, and knowledge as well as the soul. Shen/spirit guides your behaviors and actions and can be thought of as the leader of your life. Your shen/spirit is what guides you. Each person is born with shen/spirit. The elements of shen/spirit are *hún*, *pò*, *yi*, and *zhi*. I will describe these elements in detail later. The relationship between jing, qi, and shen, is very important for understanding qigong and I will describe that later too.

2. Jīng /essence is the foundation or root of life. It is each person's original good energy/yuan qi. It is stored in the kidney. Jing is a material substance that is part of the human body yet it includes substances you can see and well as those you cannot see. It is the substance that maintains life activity. It is responsible for reproduction, growth, development, and defense.

3. Xue/blood is the material substance that carries nutrients throughout the body.

4. Jīn yè / bodily fluid. Jin refers to clear fluids such as saliva, cerebral spinal fluid, etc.. Ye refers to turbid, viscous fluids. Jinye irrigates the inside of your body. For example, skin is moisturized by jinye. These fluids fill empty spaces inside ears and eyes, lubricate joints and other functions. Jinye is one of the body's three treasures.

5. Qi/energy is the driving force of life. The concept of qi has no English equivalent. The word energy is the closest English word, but it is an inadequate word to convey this important concept. Qi is a non-being substance that cannot be seen yet makes up everything in the universe. All material things result from the movement of qi. The human body is a microcosm of the universe. Qi is the driving force of the universe, each living thing, and each human. Changes in qi reflect the status of qi in a living thing. Without qi life could not exist. Qi is important in qigong since qigong adjusts qi. There are many types of qi such as body qi, wei qi, or zhen qi.

Qi drives blood flow. Each organ has its own type of qi that is characteristic of that organ.

6. Jīn Luò is a net or web of large channels (meridians) as well as a web of smaller ones. Jin luo is a control system that helps the body function. The web of jin luo channels is comparable to blood vessels because both carry nutrients. The difference is that blood vessels carry what can be seen and jin luo carry nutrients that cannot be seen except by people who have the gift of internal vision. Western physicians do not recognize internal vision as valid. Pain is caused by a lack of jin luo circulation. The circulation problem could be caused by a blockage and qigong can open these blockages. It is a pathway for blood and qi. Meridians are non-being and blood vessels are being.

Qigong/qì gōng can change your life, change your emotions. Therefore, learning qigong theory is very special. Learning about yourself is the foundation for learning about qigong because you are all you have. Understanding yourself is what is missing in western medicine. Qigong can heal the body and prevent illness from developing.

LECTURE #2
INTERNAL ORGANS *nèi zàng* & HEART

Traditional Chinese medical /zhōng yī xué thought about internal organs/*nèi zàng* is quite differently than the western medical concept of systems of organs such as the circulatory system, respiratory system, etc. The basic Chinese theory that the body must be thought of as a whole was detailed in a classic book about the body, *Zang Xiang Xue*. In Chinese medicine there are five/ wǔ zang organs in which qi "hides" or is stored. These are heart/xīn, liver/gān, spleen/pǐ , fèi/lung, and kidney/shèn . Each of these organs can be compared to a role played by the government. For example, the heart is like the emperor. There are six/liù fǔ organs which are hollow and sack-like – gall bladder/dǎn, stomach/wèi, large intestine/dà cháng, small intestine/ xiǎo cháng, bladder/páng guāng , and sān jiāo/three viscera. Zang organs are yīn and fu organs are yáng. Meridians connect all parts of the body and helps the whole body. function. Since meridians may transfer pain from a problem point to a different place in the body you must treat your whole body if you have a pain in one place.

The Chinese science has internal organs/*nèi zàng* as its basic foundation. Zang organs are the center. Channels or meridians jīng mài maintain life activity. Each zang organ works together with its corresponding fǔ organ. Jing, qi, and blood/xuè are each stored in a different organ. If each organ is filled with qi a person looks good and feels good. There are three types of organs: five zang, six fu, and "constant" organs such as the brain/nǎo, bone marrow/ suǐ , or the uterus/zi gong. The brain is connected to the kidney through the sān jiāo meridian. Every night between 9-11 then organs and this meridian receives qi from the stars.

Zang Organs – in general, these organs are for storage

1. Heart / xīn controls the passage of blood, not just in the blood vessels, also controls shen/spirit/(*hún*). The heart is like the king or emperor of the body.
2. Liver/ gān stores blood, responsible for releasing toxins, controls tendons throughout the body, opens the pupil of the eye.
3. Spleen/ pǐ guides the transport of nutrients, controls blood.
4. Lung/ fèi regulates qi, sends qi to dantian, controls water and fluid transport in the body, controls skin and hair.
5. Kidney/ shèn stores jing, controls fluids in the body in a way that is different from the lung, generates bone marrow, stores qi, opens through the ear.

Fǔ Organs – in general, these organs digest food and convert it into nutrients:

Fǔ Organs – in general, these organs digest food and convert it into nutrients

Gall bladder – dan - stores bile, helps digestion

Large intestine – da chang – transports waste

Small intestine – xiao chang – determines what is waste and what needs to be stored in the body

Stomach – wei – digests

Bladder – pang guang – stores liquid waste

San jiao – three cavities for food, air, and urine

The material above is an introduction. What follows is more detailed information.

HEART

The heart is comparable to the king or emperor of the body since it and blood control the entire body and are the engine of the body. The heart stores shen and heart qi/xin qi which is symbolized by a red bird. The heart is associated with the element fire/huǒ. I t is associated with summer. The *I Ching* / yì jīng calls it yang of yang. A normal heart beat is an indicator of a normal life. The shaoyin/heart meridian goes in three ways: down to the small intestine which is why the heart and small intestine are related, up to the eye ball, and from the heart along the inside of the arm to the tip of the little finger on both arms. Many books name only the third way, however, all three are correct.

Meridians are like highways. Blood vessels and meridians are closely related. Blood vessels can be seen, but meridians cannot. Knowledge of the meridians can help you. For example, if you cannot sleep because you are worried you can press the shenmen pressure point located on the wrist of the left hand just below the pad on the little finger side of the palm. If you have heart problems you can massage the tip of the little finger on the left hand. This works because it can remove a blockage of heart qi and blockages are the source of problems. To clear your heart and prevent heart problems place your hands on your left breast with the right hand under the left. Move your hands in a small, clockwise circle 100 times then counterclockwise 100 times. This is best done in bed immediately before sleeping.

Hǔ Yin, a Taoist physician who lived during the Tang dynasty (around 848 A.D.) had internal vision. She was a qigong grandmaster. She saw the qi of the heart is shaped like a traditional Chinese lantern. She drew a metaphorical diagram of what she saw and wrote a written description in a book titled *Wang Ting Nei Jing*. Wang ting refers to the dan zhong or middle dan dien. She drew the trigram/guà for heart, two plumes of fire, a woman, an almond shape with the radical for person/ren in it, and a red bird. The almond shape represented the soul of a person. The red bird represented a cloud of red qi that is the xīn shèn/spirit. When westerners conduct an autopsy they cannot find the red cloud of qi or the soul because they leave the body when the person dies. There is a web-like energetic covering that protects the heart using strong qi. It disappears at death.

A lot of death is caused because of ignorance of the principles and components named above. For example, tooth pain must be dealt with by adjusting the whole body. Another example is that there is a relationship between skin and body hair to the lungs so a skin problem may actually be caused by a problem in the lungs. The problem with my eyes might be due to a blockage in my heart.

When there is a problem in your body you must understand the relationships. You can learn to understand the relationships in your body over time. I am teaching Taoist theory that complements and goes beyond *The Yellow Emperor's Classic of Internal Medicine/Huang Di Nei Jing*. This information is useful in understanding the relationships in your body.

LECTURE #3 – INTERNAL ORGANS - THE LIVER

Internal organs are thought of as tissues in western medicine, however, Chinese think of internal organs differently. The Chinese character for the five internal organs/wǔ zang means five storage places. Either qi/energy or materials can be stored. Xiang is an invisible substance. It is a real substance that exists in the realm of non-being. Zang xiang xue is the main part of the study of Chinese medicine.

The liver is like an evergreen tree. The internal organ liver/ gān zang is the element of wood/ mù. Spring season is the time of the liver. It receives the growing energy of spring. It likes sour, but should be given only a little sour. The *I Ching* symbol for liver is zhèn ☳.

According to traditional Chinese medicine, the liver has many functions:

Adjusts blood supply – Liver stores blood and jing. Jing can become blood. Also, when people move around blood is transported to other organs. When people are still extra blood is stored. Thus, the liver adjusts or regulates the blood supply.

Manages qi flow – the liver can dissipate bad energy. The liver supports the stomach and spleen and digestion. Liver is "smart" at raising yang energy. At 11:00 pm, the time for gall bladder to dominate, the liver begins raising yang qi from the gall bladder and stores it for use by other organs during their time of domination (1:00-3:00 am, 3:00-5:00 am, etc.) If your abdomen feels bloated it might be because qi and blood are not being circulated well and have stagnated. Stagnation can cause tumors. Body fluid/jinye that is not circulated can produce mucus which accumulates in the blood. This is one of many possible causes of mucus. For example, mucus can be formed by issues in the lung or kidney.

Strengthens tendons (tendons and ligaments in western medicine are lumped together and called tendons in Chinese medicine) – if there is not enough blood stored in the liver then tendons might have problems. For example, there may be tingling in joints.

Adjusts emotions – When people become angry and it is controlled and released easily and naturally this does not cause a problem in the body. If people become angry and it is contained in the body for a long time energy in the liver can become bad energy.

Manages meridians – it receives qi and releases bad qi.

Hides *hún.* A fetus begins having *hún* in the third month of its development. Hun leaves the body one minute before death. Studies have been conducted that show a change in weight before and immediately after death. There are three types of *hun*: 1) tai guang is kind, helps cultivate calmness, and can determine your fate. 2) the personality who likes business and has endless greed and desire for more and more money and power. 3) guai pi is excessive, addiction to behaviors that are not open to light. Hun shapes the personality. If you cultivate virtue it and improve your hun which, in turn, improves your personality. If you know you are lacking in an area you can cultivate virtue in yourself to reduce bad and increase good aspects of *hun.* You have to change yourself instead of trying to change others. Cultivating virtue improves qigong and improving qigong improves virtue. According to ancient Chinese culture, if you are talented you act with modesty rather than showing it off or bragging about it. People who show off actually have less talent. Controls flow of fluids in the sanjiao.

If the liver has a problem there is no medicine that can cure it. The liver must be healed through healing emotions which means having an open heart, being happy, acting with kindness, and living in harmony. Since the kidney has the element water and water can help wood, having a lot of kidney energy can help heal the liver. Supporting the kidney through good nutrition can also help cure the liver.

Energy for liver comes from Jupiter/mù xīng in the east. There is a pressure point on the stomach meridian that is the entrance point for qi from Jupiter. Jing is stored mainly in the kidney, but since there is a relationship with liver, liver also stores jing.

Hu Yin, the Taoist who used her internal vision to see the energies of liver drew a metaphorical picture of what she saw just as she did for heart. The diagram includes two plumes of shen, two women, the gua for liver, a green dragon, and an image with lobes. The dragon controls how much qi is sent to each organ. Ancient Taoists also believed that the two lobes of the liver correspond to the two halves of the tai chi diagram/ tài jí tú.

LECTURE #4 – INTERNAL ORGANS – THE SPLEEN

The spleen is simpler than the heart and liver, but is it very important. Spleen is the central control mechanism in the body.

Hua Yin drew a diagram of the spleen illustrating what she saw using her internal vision just as she did for the heart and liver. The diagram had a yellow phoenix, two plumes depicting the soul, and the bagua diagram for earth.

According to traditional Chinese medicine, the spleen has multiple functions:

Combining nutrients and chemicals from food then transporting them to the blood and other organs (especially heart and lungs)

Balance Water – the body is composed mostly of water, extra water is used by the spleen to help with transport. The spleen and lungs work together to balance water.

Spleen controls the direction of movement of blood in vessels including the capillaries.

Spleen problems or weaknesses can manifest on the skin. This is because a weak spleen leaves too much dampness in the body. The external opening of spleen is the lips. If the lips are too white or too purple it is an indication of a spleen problem. There is often a relationship with the heart and lungs for passing blood from the spleen to the lung. If your spleen is good then lungs are helped.

In the five elements, spleen is represented by earth. The planet earth in the universe parallels the spleen in the body. Earth contributes wood to fire. Fire contributes to earth. The spleen is near the middle portion of the *sanjiao*.

Spleen hides yi which is intention and intellect/memory. Yi is also called zhen qi. It is present at birth and can be cultivated during life. The brain gets zhen qi from the spleen. Because spleen is so involved with intellect and intention, too much worry and mental rumination can damage the spleen. Happiness nourishes the spleen. Clearing the mind during qigong helps the spleen. Saturn is the planet related to spleen. Qi from Saturn begins growing in June. 9 – 11 am is the time of spleen.

Zang organs produce medicines within the body. Organs help each other by radiating qi to each other. There is a relationship between organs and the universe. There are deep mathematical formulas about the interactions among organs, but it is very deep and I will not explain these.

August 8 is the beginning of the fall season. Eighteen days before the start of each season the spleen is dominant. Eating at night is not good for the spleen because it continues to work during a period when it could be resting.

Every organ stores shen.

Barley soup is good for spleen. Since there is a relationship between spleen and skin, barley soup can help itchy skin.

LECTURE #5 – INTERNAL ORGANS – LUNGS

Lung is very important and its functions are complicated. Most lung function happens in the right lung because of the space occupied by the heart.

Inhale natural qi, exhale bad qi. The Chinese understanding of inhaling and exhaling is different and more complex than the western understanding. In Chinese philosophy, the body receives qi through a) inhalation and b) consumption of food. Lungs relate to the spleen in the details of using food and drink. The spleen sends good qi from food to the lungs where it is combined with inhaled natural qi to form *zong qi*. *Zong qi* is formed from *ying*/nutritional qi and protective/*wei qi*. *Ying qi* is inside both small and large meridians. *Wei qi* is outside meridians.

Distribution of body qi/*zong qi*. Ying qi goes to internal organs from the lungs. Wei qi is also formed from nutrition gained through food, however; it functions to protect the body and especially the skin. The lung can be compared to the shifu of an emperor because it determines how much *zong qi* is needed by each internal organ. The spleen assists in the distribution of *zong qi* to internal organs. Yuan qi/original qi depends on zong qi to maintain life. The *san jiao* has original/*yuan qi* which is the qi with which each person is born. The lung sends yuan qi to the *san jiao* where it assists with metabolism.

Controls movement of water and bodily fluids/jin ye through the body and down to the kidney as well as how much water is lost through sweat and through exhalation. Useful parts of water are recirculated in the body and waste water is made into urine in the kidneys. Lungs, kidneys, and spleen are all involved in the movement of fluid, however, lungs are the main mover. When fluids leave the body they carry bad qi outside the body. If the lungs do not circulate water well then high blood pressure can result.

There is a complex relationship between humans and the universe. The Chinese calendar has twenty-four parts called *jie ji*. Meridians have connections to the *jie ji*. Lungs connect the organs via meridians. The stomach meridian passes through the knee so if stomach qi is not good it effects lung qi. Another example is the human knee which has twenty-four bones in traditional Chinese medicine. These correspond to the twenty-four *jie ji*. Chinese believe it is best if a baby does not practice walking for a full year after birth because it can damage the knee and lungs. The lung is closely related to the large intestine. Fall is the time to strengthen lungs. It is best to get up early in the fall. Adjusting breathing during qigong is particularly important during the fall because it is the time for clearing the lungs so they perform their functions effectively.

I mentioned in a previous lecture that *hún* hides in/is stored in the liver. Pò is associated with the lung. Western psychology has the concepts of rationality and instinct that are somewhat similar to *hun* and *po* although there are some important differences between rationality and its Chinese comparison *hun* as well as between instinct and *po*. There are seven types of *po* and each is a different type of qi. They are extremely difficult to describe in English. One type of *po* is excessive desire for money. The calmer you are the more this type of po is diminished. What is key is that western psychology defines the soul as having rational and instinctual components. In Chinese thought each of the seven aspects has characteristics that are embedded in the *po* soul. Excessive desire is an example of one of the seven. Each person has varying amounts of each of the seven. Like *hun*, unhelpful characteristics can be diminished through cultivating virtue in one's life.

Hun and *po* are invisible, non-being substances. *Hun* can be compared to the main part of the soul and *po* to a smaller part. *Po* is related to your personality. One type of *po* removes impurities and contaminants from inhaled air. *Po* is in the right side of the lung. *Hun* enters the fetus at three months and *po* enters at four months. *Hun* leaves the body through the mouth and bei hui immediately before death. *Po* leaves through the anus after death. It can take as long as forty-nine days after death for *po* to leave. Although the body is dead, death is not complete until the po leaves.

Hu Yin drew a diagram of lung that has seven people to represent the seven types of *po*. There is also a white tiger that represents lung shen and lung qi. A group of fourteen singers represents a chorus of fourteen who sing at a very high pitch. Some people can hear this music during qigong. The direction for lung is west. It's star is Venus.

LECTURE #6 – INTERNAL ORGANS – KIDNEY

Jing is the original energy/*yuan qi*. It is the driving force of the body. It is given by the parents. The Chinese radical for qi contains the radical for rice. Rice and other food inside the body becomes nutritive qi. The radical for jing also contains the radical for rice. Rice being part of the radical for qi and jing shows the importance of food qi.

Hair is "the flower" of the kidney. It reflects the health of the kidney. The aspect of *shen* known as *zhi* is related to ambition so if the kidney has lots of qi you are highly motivated. Someone with strong kidneys will have lots of saliva. Qigong increases the amount of saliva. There is a relationship between kidneys and the ears and the urethra. There is also a relationship with sexual activity. The kidney works with the bladder to condense qi to form water. The development of an embryo begins at the kidney. Original jing is stored in the kidney. The amount of *jing* (also called *jing qi*) with which you are born influences the length of your life. A lot of *jing* means a long life unless you spend too much or let too much drain away.

Spending *jing qi* or allowing it to drain away shortens your life. Conserving *jing qi* lengthens your life. Clearing your kidney lengths your life because it helps jing qi. Adults who have too much sex drain their jing qi. Young boys have a lot of *jing qi* so draining it is not a concern. Eating too much ice cream or drinking icy drinks drains *jing qi*. This is because the body maintains a constant temperature, however, consuming ice cream or icy drinks requires spending jing qi to adjust for the coldness to maintain the body's normal temperature. Both western and Chinese medicines can have the effect of creating coldness in the body and can damage your liver or your original qi/*yuan qi* so it is advisable to take the smallest amount of medicine possible.

The kidney sends nutrition to the brain. If you do not have enough kidney qi you may have low intelligence or may become confused easily. 3:00-5:00 p.m. is the time of the bladder. If you are frequently tired during this time of day you may not have enough qi. 5:00-7:00 p.m. is the time of the kidney.

Kidney and the Universe

People with internal vision have seen that the Milky Way is energetically connected to the kidney. Energy to the kidney is strong in winter so this is a good time to clear the kidney. Mercury is the planet associated with kidney. The *mingmen* (ming = life, men = door . . . mingmen = door of life) is connected to the universe and they exchange qi. People with internal vision universe and kidney together form a yin-yang symbol/*tai chi tu*. The *Dao De Jing* has a phrase that refers to the *mingmen* (ping), (this was not translated into English). Yang starts at winter solstice. Spinal fluid is related to the mingmen and spine. Yin and yang are strong in original qi/yuan qi. The mingmen reflects through the eyes. Hu Yin's diagram to represent what she saw with her internal vision has a two-headed deer, but in winter is becomes a snake and turtle.

The *Yellow Emperor's Classic of Internal Medicine/Huang Di Nei Jing* describes *Xing* and ming. *Xing* is spiritual in nature and is the site of *shen*, *yi*, *hun*, *po*, and *zhi*. Ming is life. Buddha cultivated xing. Taoists cultivate both *xing* and *ming*.

Cultivating calm protects the kidney. A calm person tends to live a long life. Strong, loud music heard for a long time consumes jing qi which shortens life.

Kidney doesn't cause pain when there's a problem. Instead, it causes tiredness. Kidney is crucial because weak kidney can cause problems in the heart or lung. If your body is tired every day even if you take a nap or do qigong it may be an indicator of problems with your kidney or spleen. The tiredness could be your body's way of telling you there is a problem with kidney. Kidney problems result in tiredness in the afternoon, spleen or lung problems result in waking up tired.

LECTURE #7 – FU ORGANS – GALL BLADDER

The study of internal organs is called *zang xiang xue*. There is a close relationship between qigong and understanding the internal organs – five *zang* organs have already been subjects of lectures. *Zang* organs (liver, heart, spleen, lungs, kidneys) are solid organs that store *jing, qi, shen, hun* (liver), and *po* (lung). *Jing* can be seen sometimes since it forms bodily fluids *(jin ye)*. Today is the first lecture on fu organs. *Fu* organs gall bladder, stomach, small intestine, large intestine, bladder, san jiao) are even more important than zang. 2/3 of the universe and 2/3 of the human body are non-being. *Fu* organs are comparable to non-being. *Dao De Jing* (chapter 11) is about the importance of empty spaces. An empty room is more important than the walls because the empty space can be used. *Fu* organs have empty space that can be used.

The gall bladder starts a small fire that grows throughout the twelve two-hour periods of the day. It is comparable like the rat which is the first of twelve signs of the Chinese zodiac. It can also be compared to a key being put into the ignition of a car to start the engine. The heart is the engine. If the gall bladder is weak the heart tends to be weak. The kidney is like the fuel tank of a car. A car works well if it has oil. *Yuan qi* could be compared to oil.

Functions of the Gall Bladder:

1. Generate bile. Bile has qi from the liver. If the liver is strong then the bile is strong. Bile assist the small intestine. Bile is yellow.

2. Help judgment and courage. An individual can look at a problem in a helpful or unhelpful way. Gall bladder qi can help you become calm during difficult times. When catastrophe strikes, a person with a strong gall bladder can deal more effectively. If a person's emotions are not good it could be because the gall bladder is weak.

3. Junction of yin and yang in the body. This is very complicated and will be described later.

Signs of a weak gall bladder:

1. Saliva tastes bitter when you awaken in the morning
2. Sighing frequently for no reason at all and emotions are not involved
3. Pain in the outside corner of the eye
4. Pain in top of neck where meridian passes through

Improve gall bladder by:

1. Sleeping between 11:00 p.m. and 1:00 a.m. because this is the time gall bladder does its work. Sleeping at other times does not make up for the support for the gall bladder that occurs when sleeping during these hours.
2. Eating a healthy breakfast
3. Eating on a consistent schedule
4. Avoiding stress
5. Chewing food well
6. Avoiding dry food

LECTURE #8 – FU ORGANS – STOMACH

Functions of the Stomach:

1. Receive food. The stomach becomes an "ocean" of water and food. Nutrients are taken from food and water. Lung qi needs nutrients from food.
2. Move nutrients to spleen which sends them to other organs
    a. Pathway #1 from spleen - transports nutrients to the heart and lungs.
    b. Pathway #2 from spleen - transports nutrients to the small intestines which extracts physical nutrients. Then, large intestines remove any remaining nutrients before elimination of waste.
3. Collect qi from constellations to send to kidneys. The kidney is symbolized by turtle, black, winter. Other stars also send qi the the stomach. (White rabbit in fall ????)

Between 7:00 – 9:00 p.m. yang qi is fully present.

Signs of a weak stomach:

1. Sensitive startle response
2. Yawning
3. Cold sores on the mouth

4. Blackish color on the face or a face that is white

5. Ache in the teeth of the upper jaw

Improve stomach by eating a breakfast that is nutritious, not necessarily delicious between 7:00 a.m. – 9:00 a.m. which is the time for stomach. It continues the increase of the flame that is started by the gall bladder. Good food during this time is precious like a spring drizzle. At breakfast, it is okay to eat to 90% full. Eating later in the day should only be to 70% full. Lunch is also a time for nutritious food and is the best time to eat meat. Once yin starts to build at noon it is better not to eat meat. Dinner should be the lightest meal.

LECTURE #9 – FU ORGANS – SMALL INTESTINE

Functions:

1. Holds food for a small amount of time so food can be digested beyond that done in the stomach. Once this digestion is complete it is assimilated and transformed into jing qi.

2. Separates good (clear) and bad fluid (murky)then transfers nutrients to the spleen and nutritious fluid and jing are sent to the spleen (good) and kidney (waste). Spleen then sends good water to lungs.

3. Transfers jing qi to organs

4. Sends waste to proper organ. Fluid waste to kidney and bladd, solid waste to large intestine

5. Creates yao, a natural medicine that is an even more refined nutrient that is removed from food, then uses it to assist organs

Symptoms of Problems:

1. Blood in urine
2. Dry tongue
3. Sleep difficulties
4. Pain in teeth in upper jaw
5. Swollen abdomen
6. Hearing problems
7. Jaundiced eye (also symptom of gall bladder problems)

Too much heart fire can cause intestinal problems because the meridians for heart and small intestine are close to one another and so there is a relationship. An example is that stress causes heart fire which causes chronic diarrhea.

To help small intestine

1. Foods – millet, congee, soupy foods
2. Chew food well before swallowing

LECTURE #10 – FU ORGANS – LARGE INTESTINE

Functions:

1. Absorb nutrients from food and release waste
2. Receives remaining water after small intestine does its work then transforms the water in jin ye (sweat, saliva, tears, urine, etc.

Symptoms of Problems:

1. Constant sweating even when not exercising
2. Diarrhea (nutrients are lost)
3. Very large neck
4. Sounds in the ear (symptomatic of insufficient amount of jin ye)
5. Pain in vicinity of large intestine meridian (abdomen, upper arms, lower jaw)

Hŭ Yin used her gift of internal vision and saw light coming from a "star" to the intestine. The light formed a circle in the abdomen that was white at the beginning then changed to other colors throughout the length of the small intestine then was black at the end. The appendix has a pressure point that is a direct connection to the start for large intestine.

LECTURE #11 – FU ORGANS – BLADDER

The lung is the origin of water in the body. It sends water to the spleen which, in turn, sends it to the bladder. These three organs have a relationship through which qi is transformed. This relationship will become clearer in lecture twelve which will be about the sān jiāo.

Functions

1. Stores water from stomach and spleen for a short time, transforms it to urine which is excreted.

2. Stores water from stomach and spleen for a short time, transforms it to varied forms of jin ye then distributes it to areas of need. Nutrients remaining in water are removed and transformed into jin ye before urine is formed. This storage is in a sac within the bladder.

Symptoms of Problems:

1. Dry skin can be from insufficient *jin ye*
2. Insufficient saliva
3. Headache
4. Tension in the back
5. Waist pain
6. Leg cramps
7. Heaviness of legs can mean problems in bladder have spread to kidney.

Ways to Promote Health of Bladder:

1. Bladder meridian (called sun meridian) which goes up the back of the leg from the small toes, up both sides of spine and up to back of head is very important. Exposing your back to the sun is good for this meridian

2. Stretching your legs can open the meridian and improve circulation.

3. Soaking feet in hot water can open the meridian and improve circulation.

LECTURE #12 – FU ORGANS – SAN JIAO

The *sān jiāo*, one of the six hollow/fu organs, is a very important organ. An ancient book titled *Zhong Zang Jing* provides information about the *sān jiāo*. It is an invisible organ with no physical shape which means it is Non-Being. The three lines on the left portion of this character represent three. The top portion of the right side of the character represents a bird and the lower portion represents a small fire. The two parts of the right side symbolize roasting a chicken over a small fire. There is no good English equivalent for *sān jiāo*, but the best is Triple Warmer since the left side represents three and the right side represents roasting a chicken. The right side can also be thought of as browning something in an oven.

The *sān jiāo* can be thought of in two ways. The less common usage is big sān jiāo/da sān jiāo which includes the whole body. In the da sān jiāo the three portions are from the neck up, the torso, and legs and feet. The most common usage of sān jiāo includes only the torso. In this usage, the upper jiāo/shang jiao is the chest, the middle jiāo/zhong jiao is the upper abdomen, and the lower jiāo/xia jiao is the lower abdomen. Each to jiāo is associated with organs of the body. The upper jiāo is associated with the heart and lungs. The middle jiāo is associated with the spleen, stomach, gall bladder, and liver. The lower jiāo is associated with the intestines, kidney, and the bladder.

Functions:

1. Clears meridians throughout the body
2. Delivers *yuan qi* from the kidney to *fu* and *zang* organs as *jin ye* and water.
3. Transforms nutrients from food into qi.
4. Fosters a relationship among all organs, the five elements, and muscles and tendons.

In 2008, a 50 year old Daoist who had internal vision began an intense three month study of the activity of the *san jiao*. Using this vision he could see that there is a two-hour period between nine and 11:00 PM during which the *sān jiāo* the exchanges qi with the big universe. He watched the entire two hours and saw that during this time the *sān jiāo* cycles qi from the universe through the body five times.

18 SEASONAL HEALTH PRACTICES

The Chinese health culture focuses on prevention of illness by living in ways that contribute to balancing yin and yang in the body. Each human is a miniature universe that corresponds to the large universe. Yin and yang are constantly going in and out of balance in both. The cycles of the human body are closely related to the cycle of the seasons; therefore, it is desirable to adjust food, clothing, exercise, sleep, and sexual activity to imitate changes with the seasons to promote internal balance. This is called following the flow of the universe.

In nature and in our bodies there are five elements that interact in creative and destructive cycles. The five elements are wood, fire, earth, air, and water. As the cycles in our bodies change as we move through the seasons we must adjust our habits of eating, sleeping, sex, and exercise to have the maximum benefit from the energy of the seasons. The body changes in response to food, weather, time of day which makes it important to follow nature to help the body.

It takes a long time to become ill and a long time before symptoms show. Healing takes a long time too. Medicine gives the appearance of healing, but true healing takes a long time. Disease can be caused externally by atmospheric influences and internally by excess emotions. The six atmospheric influences which are sometimes translated as evil influences are wind, cold, summer heat, fire, dampness, and dryness. If they follow change of weather as normal through the year then it is okay. When they don't exist in the normal sequence the imbalance makes people more vulnerable to sickness. Emotions and the body are closely linked especially joy, anger, worry, anxiety, sadness or grief, and fear. Normal levels of emotion are not harmful, however, high intensity emotions that last a long time can damage internal organs – too much joy harms the heart, too much worry damages the spleen, sadness the lung, fear the kidney, and anger the liver. Stagnation of qi can be caused by many things such as stress, anger, sadness, some foods, toxins, weather. Joy can be understood as happiness, kindness, or peacefulness. Americans do not differentiate between worry anxiety and fear anxiety.

Caring for yourself in one season by eating good food and being active yet not too active improves your health in the next. Adjusting your lifestyle choices to follow the seasonal changes in the universe will help protect you against challenges from external influences. Controlling your emotions will minimize the effect of excess emotions on your body. General principles for making helpful lifestyle choices are summarized below followed by details that are specific to each season. If your body does not have enough *yin qi* or *yang qi* the deficiency can be made up with proper food, tai chi, and qigong. Each person is different and different bodies can need different foods. The guidelines below are generalized and may need to be tailored to the specific needs of an individual.

Food and Drink

Your food needs to change regularly because the yin and yang in your body changes every day so you should eat a wide variety of food to support your body in adjusting to the changes. Breakfast should be high quality. Lunch should be high in quantity and include meat. Dinner should be a low quantity. Eating grain and vegetables at a meal is important as is eating a bit of meat. Meat that has some fat is best because your body needs oil and fat is a place where energy is stored. Fruit cannot be the main food at a meal because it is not "solid" like grain.

It is best if the food you eat changes along with changes in the universe. There are general guidelines for what to eat in each season, however, each person is different so the diet must be adjusted according to individual needs. For example, a person with less fire than most people should not attempt to cool fire as much as most people. Balance in eating is key. Consuming quality food and being selective about what you eat and drink is important for promoting your health. Avoid what is not good for your body even if it is your favorite. Also avoid junk, canned, deep fried, and fatty foods as well as food containing additives or growth hormones. Processed foods are convenient, but bad for your body. Avoid eating within three hours of bedtime. Eating soupy meals for breakfast and dinner and solid food at lunch is best. Steaming foods is healthiest.

The more you do qigong the more selective you need to become about what you eat. For example, your body will not tolerate some foods any longer such as greasy, fried food. Avoid overuse of microwave ovens because radiation protections built into the ovens they filter most, but not all of the radiation.

Overeating even what is good is not good. Eating too much at one time is problem can cause stomach and possibly small intestine problems. Eating soup at the beginning of a meal can help you avoid over eating. Eating to seventy percent full is ideal. Western scientists experiments with monkeys and after ten years those that were fed to full at every meal had higher cholesterol and many physical problems. Those fed to only seventy percent full were healthier and longer lived. Humans need a diet that is approximately thirty percent protein.

Grains and Beans

Chinese believe baked goods are not good for you. Rice that sticks to pan and burns is not good. When you toast, let it cool down a bit. Mung bean soup will clear your internal organs. It will calm itching. Adding millet to mung bean soup increases the nutritional value. Adding dried bulb from a lily flower increases the nutrition even more. In China, women eat millet soup for the first two months after giving birth to increase milk production and to promote sleep.

Vegetables

Examples of vegetables that fall within the colors associated with the five elements are 1) Green – kiwi which helps prevent cancer and hardening of arteries, celery, cucumber, 2) Red – tomato, little red wine with dinner, radish, 3) Yellow – carrots, yams, corn, pumpkin, squash, 4) White – daikon radish, fresh garlic which is best when eaten raw after being cut into small pieces and let sit for fifteen minutes and 5) Black – eggplant, dried Chinese mushroom, seaweed such as kombu or nori. Onions are good for bones

Fruits and Nuts

No information about fruits and nuts in general was given.

Meat and Fish

It is helpful to limit meat because it has an acidic nature while increasing alkaline foods such as vegetables.

Other Foods

Oil for cooking changes in a bad way if it gets above 300 degrees. Olive oil is good to eat. Cold pressed is preferable because it has not lost nutrients in processing. Ginger is very good for some people, but not for others. For most people a little ginger is good every day, but too much makes fire and is bad for eyes. If a person has too much yang then eating ginger is good because it's hot. Ginger with meat or fish is good. Cutting ginger finely makes it spicier/hotter.

Beverages

Drink at least eight cups of good quality water or tea daily. Tea should be made fresh daily. Green tea in morning is beneficial. Don't drink distilled water because it becomes acidic. Drinking water before a meal aids digestion.

Clothing

Wearing clothes of one hundred percent cotton is preferable to wearing unnatural fibers.

Exercise and Qigong

Daily exercise is important; however, take care to balance activity and rest. Consider what is good for cultivating both yin and yang. Too much exercise depletes yang while too little exercise causes qi and blood to stagnate. American culture is very yang so Americans have tendency to overdo yang when exercising. Tai chi chuan[1] is a form of aerobic exercise. The traditional Yang style 118 long form takes twenty-five to thirty minutes and opens cells, causes sweating, is very healthy and safe. Other types of exercise are okay as play. Americans often exercise in closed buildings; however, that is not the Chinese way. Walking outside is better than inside on a treadmill. Chlorine in swimming pools is bad.

Practicing both tai chi and qigong contributes to balance by linking the mind and body and coordinating the working of the internal organs. Thirty to sixty minutes of tai chi and qigong in whatever

The pinyin spelling is taiji quan or taijiquan and the Wade-Giles spelling is t'ai chi ch'uan.

outward. Yin and yang become balanced. During qigong energy similar to an electric current goes to any place needing healing and breaks stagnant energy. Qigong is a way to heal yourself. Doing qigong will connect mind and body in healthy ways that conform to the natural state of the universe. During qigong excess emotions leave the body. For example, crying can release sadness that has been stored in the lung. People who practice tai chi and qigong come back into balance at higher and higher levels.

Sleep

Although everyone needs a different amount of sleep it is best not sleep more than nine hours a day and not less than four. Sleeping on your side is better than on your back because it conserves energy. Use blankets made of natural materials rather than electric ones. Wool is best. Down is satisfactory yet less desirable because the small feathers of down feathers may bother older adults. Also, minimize the amount of electronic equipment in your bedroom and do not have a television in your bedroom.

Sexual Activity

No general guidelines were described. This is a very deep subject and only general information was provided in class.

Emotions

It is important to maintain positive, balanced emotions. Start everyday thinking it will be a good day and smile. The physical act of smiling initiates physiological changes that impact emotions. Practice smiling at least three times a day when you are alone. Laughing hard at least three times a day will contribute to a long life. There are studies that show that people who laugh a lot are healthy and less prone to overweight. When you are sad crying releases sad feelings out. It is easier for women to cry than men who are trained to keep it inside. Men need to learn from women and need to release emotion. Some excess emotions can be released by talking about what is bothersome.

SPRING SEASON

Spring is the most important season to take care of yourself. The element for spring is wood color is green, direction is east. Spring is a time of volatile changes in the weather and rapid shifts between warm temperatures in daytime and cold at night. During this season it can be quite windy. Prevent wind from entering the body by wearing enough clothing. Spring wind sometimes has good energy, sometimes bad. Germs are more and more active as the earth warms and the Universe comes back to life. These intense changes stress the human body and make it more vulnerable to illness. The lungs are a doorway to the body so it is important to keep your chest warm in the spring to protect it from the effects of bad energy. The sān jiāo [2] is near the lungs and must be protected from bad energy. Joint and heart problems are most likely to manifest in spring. Old health problems recur more easily in spring than the rest of the year. When the second half of Chinese spring starts the vulnerability decreases.

In spring, the element is wood relating in our bodies to the liver. At this time there is lot of energy to heal the liver and it is important to keep that energy in balance. There is more and more *yang qi* as the season progresses. It goes to the liver, but sometimes you need yang lower in your body in the kidneys. The liver, like wood, is vulnerable to fire which humans experience as angry feelings if the energy in the liver becomes too hot.

In each season opposite conditions exist in the body from what exists in nature. In spring it is becoming warmer outside yet the inside of the body is still cold inside in the early spring and must be protected from coldness. This is especially important in years when it takes a long time for the weather to warm up. The weather is volatile and the fluctuations that are typical in spring increase vulnerability to colds and flu.

If you take care of yourself now, you will be stronger the rest of the year. Spring is for clearing the liver and increasing yang qi. Yang qi

[2] There is no adequate English equivalent of san jiao even though it is often translated into English as Triple Warmer or Triple Burner.

begins to increase in the spring and growth starts in nature and in the human body. The body grows in energy just like the flowers and other plants grow in the spring. In spring your body needs to receive yang. You can take advantage of the increase in yang qi in this season by practicing tai chi, Five Elements, ma bu, and qigong outside during good weather as soon as it is warm enough and as long as it is not windy. If the liver is strong the spleen and stomach will be stronger. Caring for the spleen and stomach results in caring for the liver. If your liver energy is good, enough then you'll be energetic. If not enough, you'll be tired, not enough energy to do what you want.

Chinese tradition makes recommendations for promoting your health during the spring. They are particularly beneficial for the stomach which, in turn, benefits the liver. Swish water inside your mouth upon waking and after eating. Spit the water out after swishing. Click teeth together thirty-six times after waking in the morning. Do thirty-six hand circles on your abdomen after waking in the morning. Spend three minutes looking far away to look at trees or other parts of nature. Paying attention to the green is particularly helpful. Slowly walk about one hundred paces after eating a meal.

Jin jou is the 3rd part of spring season. This is an easy time to have high blood pressure or heart problems so be careful to clear your heart. It is particularly important to balance yin and yang in a way that parallels the yin and yang in the universe. This is a good time to do tai chi and standing qigong outside if it is not windy. Do sitting qigong inside. Eat foods that are not too hot, not too cold. Wear clothes to stay warm regardless of changes in weather. This is an easy time for stroke or high blood pressure.

Gou yu/grain rain is the last of the two-week periods of the spring. It is typically a time of rain. It will soon start to warm, but it is still cool in this period so continue wearing enough clothes to stay warm. Once in the 18-day period before the start of summer it is good to clear the spleen

Food and Drink

Choose foods for their health value rather than because they are delicious. Consume a wide variety of foods with a focus on those that support the liver. Avoid heavy foods. Watery soup is highly recommended, but not American soups with salt and cream. Bean or vegetable soups are best. Chicken soup is okay unless you have high blood pressure. Cooking a Cornish hen stuffed with dates in water for about an hour is good to eat three or four times a week to increase energy. Ginseng can be used in soup to increase energy. Ginseng grown in America is weak and can be used by anyone. Ginseng grown in China or Korea where it grows naturally is very strong and should be used only to help sick people. Congee is also good in spring. Minimize food and drink that is cold. Warm food and drink is best. Consumption of cold items can damage the stomach while items that are extremely hot because it can damage the lining of the stomach. Do not force yourself to eat or drink. Inability to find any food that is appealing is a sign that the stomach is not well and that *wei qi* may be deficient. If you do not have *wei qi* you will die.

Grains and Beans

Eat a wide variety of grains whether you enjoy them or not. All grains can be eaten in spring; however, barley and millet are the best grains in this season. White rice can be eaten once or twice a week. Yellow, black, soy, and mung beans are recommended in spring. Beans are good if you cook them a long time and cook them yourself. It's easy! Put them in boiling water, when water returns to a boil, turn heat down to simmer for twenty to thirty minutes. Tofu is good except if you have circulation problems. Dates and goji berries and good spring choices especially in soup. Avoid brown rice because it is more difficult to digest. Avoid lily flour in the spring. This is made by grinding dried lily flower buds. Fresh lily has toxins do not eat it ever.

Vegetables

Increase consumption of vegetables. Green vegetables are best especially spinach which should always be eaten cooked which removes damaging oxalic acid. Avoid eating spinach with tofu because eating them together creates unhealthy chemicals. Sprouts of mung bean and soy bean are also beneficial in spring. Red radishes and daikon radishes are beneficial unless they upset your stomach. Celery, cucumbers, sweet potatoes, and raw garlic are beneficial in spring. Lots of roughage promotes healthy functioning of bowels. The first spring crop of garlic chives has a lot of yang.

Fruits, Nuts, and Seeds

Apples, kiwi, papaya, banana, grapefruit, and pineapples are beneficial in spring. Apricots, nectarines, mango, pears, and tangerines can increase liver fire so consumption of these fruits should be minimal. Sesame seeds are a useful addition to the diet this time of year. Black have more nutrition than white. Goji berries and red dates help clear the liver of toxins.

Meat and Fish

Eating less meat, fat, and oil at this time of year helps keep the liver in balance. Eating some meat is acceptable. Eating meat at lunchtime is preferable to eating it for dinner. The World Health Organization labels duck as a high-quality protein and it is fine to eat in spring. Eat any kind of meat except lamb which is a warming food which should be eaten in winter not spring since it can result in too much internal fire. Intake of chicken and turkey should be minimized in spring. Fish eaten this time of year will create mucus if you have a cold or other sickness. Fish from the ocean is better than fresh water fish in springtime. Meat will cause much fire if eaten when you are ill.

Other Foods

In terms of spices, some salt is okay in spring as is a little sugar. The spleen likes sweet and the spleen supports the liver which means supporting the spleen helps the liver. A small amount of chocolate is okay. The liver likes sour and some sour such as vinegar or lemon is very good for the liver, but too much keeps yang from rising. Also, too much sour will stress spleen which, in turn, taxes the stomach. If your liver is not strong, a bit of sweet such as a small amount of dark chocolate can be helpful. Too much salt is bad for your kidneys. MSG is bad for your body and should never be eaten. Cayenne and hot peppers can make fire.

Beverages

Drink lots of water with or without lemon and avoid sweet drinks including fruit juice. Drinking too much water at once is not good for the stomach.

Clothing

Paying careful attention to your choices in clothing is important to be sure you are warm enough. The weather in spring is not cold enough to freeze water, but cold enough to "freeze" people. Avoid the temptation to shed clothes early in the season just because a particular day is warm. It is important to continue to dress warmly including wearing socks, shoes rather than sandals, and a hat. After the first two parts of spring season it is warm enough to begin wearing less clothing. Keeping your head warm is important so continue wearing a hat because the breezes can be chilly. Keeping your feet warm is also important so wear shoes, not sandals and no bare feet. Women must be more careful than men to protect the abdomen and waist. This can be done by keeping the legs warm by wearing pants rather than skirts. Hair should be worn loose and natural rather than being bound. Clothes should be loose. After the fourth two-week period of spring, *qin ming* it is okay to begin wearing less clothes.

Exercise and Qigong

Although too much exercise is not good in spring season, exercise is important for maintaining flexibility. Exercising early in the morning, outside if weather permits, enhances receipt of the yang energy that increases in the spring. Do not do heavy exercise after eating.

Doing qigong and tai chi daily is particularly important in the spring. Practicing one in the morning and one in the evening is good. As your body becomes stronger by doing qigong over a long period of time then your immune system is stronger and will not be impacted as much by spring changes in nature. Increase the amount of tai chi over what you do in winter. Doing tai chi will keep your tendons from tightening. Be sure to leave time between qigong and tai chi. There is a close relationship between the liver and eyes so if your eyes water or your nose runs during qigong it can mean fire is being released from your liver.

Sleep

The sun rises earlier as the days begin to lengthen in spring and it is natural to wake up earlier and go to bed earlier. A lot of sleep is needed this time of year. Six to eight hours of sleep is good. Being asleep by 11:00 pm and rising early is a useful guideline. It is important to get up early because it helps awaken yang energy. Being asleep between 1:00-3:00 am is important since this is the most important time of day for clearing the liver. If you are tired in the afternoon, take a nap for thirty minutes or less. Too much sleep at this time is bad for the tendons of the body.

Sexual Activity

During this yang time, it is natural to have more sex than in the winter. Twice a week is a good balance for most people. Having too much sex or other physical activity can deplete *jing* which is the life energy found in the fluids of the body such as spinal fluid, saliva, and reproductive fluids. The best time for sexual activity is 8pm-midnight. Jing is stored in the kidney. Practicing qigong can replenish jing, but it is best to keep all activities in balance and not deplete it in the first place.

It is important that both partners feel good after sex and that they treat each other with kindness and respect. The quality of sexual relations can affect future generations. Avoid having sex when you are angry or drunk. Conceiving a baby when angry or after drinking too much alcohol is unhealthy for the baby.

Emotions

The weather in spring is changeable and so are emotions. It is easy to become worried or angry during spring. When you are angry the level of your good energy is low and immunity weakens. If you're angry for more than five minutes toxins begin to develop that can damage the liver and negatively impact the rest of the body because it interferes with the flow of energy in the liver meridians. A major liver meridian goes from the toe up to the head and crosses at the eyeball so anger is not good for the eyes. When you are angry yang rises in your body and can cause problems in the brain such as headache or stroke. It is particularly important to avoid anger in the morning and after a meal.   .

Clearing your liver will help keep your emotions from getting too strong. Learn to control your emotions and to keep yourself from becoming angry. If someone is angry at you try not to get upset. Avoid letting other people's anger hurt you. You will be better able to do this if your liver is balanced. The longer you do qigong the more you'll be able to control your own feelings and you will not easily anger when someone else is angry.   If you have a bad temper then do something to change the angry feeling. Complaining is not good for you. It generates anger and keeps it going. Instead, you should release bad energy and become calm. When you experience short term such as anger at a family member release it by talking about it, listening to music, imagining a bright clear light inside you or holy water showering you and entering you through the top of your head and cleaning you internally, or doing whatever helps you get over it. If you are angry and cannot let it go then go for a walk until the anger is gone. Thinking about the cause of anger will not help. If the anger is over a long time such as anger at the government it needs to be released. Try talking about it with good friends about the problems you see. It might help you to discover solutions or ways to melt the anger. If you cannot find a group in which to talk then find other ways to release the anger. Be careful who you pick, because if you select people with bad energy then it can end up hurting you rather than helping.

Other

At night during any time of the year, soak your feet in hot water for twenty minutes. Make the water deep enough to cover your ankles and up to the knees, if possible. Add hot water as necessary to keep the water hot. This is beneficial because your feet have many meridians. Water hotter than 130^0 F can disrupt your sleep so don't make it any hotter than this.

SUMMER SEASON

Chinese philosophy developed over time through observation of the natural world. Summer has a yang nature and yang energy is abundant. On the day after summer solstice yin starts to build and the dominate *Yi Jing/I Ching* hexagram shifts from ☰☰ to ☰☰. Everything is growing to its peak. Bodily metabolism of humans is at its most active. The day before summer solstice is the day that has the most yang. On the day of solstice all things that are yang in nature begin to decline, but plants that possess yin nature flourish more. Eat noodles on the summer solstice and dumplings or pancakes on the winter solstice. Deer's antler grown less after solstice. Cicadas buzz after solstice because they have yin nature.

In terms of five elements, summer is the time of fire. It is time to clear and care for heart. At this time of year humans are hot on the outside, yet cold on the inside so your body needs warmth inside. Avoid cold draughts. Drinking warm beverages or eating hot soup will help bad energy go out of the body as does eating kiwi or watermelon. Eating or drinking cold foods feels good at the time; however, it exacerbates the cold on the inside. Internal cold can damage your internal organs. Dampness drawn into the body can stress the kidney. Swimming is fine, but when you are resting the dampness can be drawn into the body easily so it is best to avoid sitting on rocks, damp sand at the beach, and wet benches for a long time. Sleeping on cool stone has the same effect. Fresh air is much more healthy than air conditioning. Too much dampness produces internal fire. If your saliva is bitter it is a sign of too much fire which is bad for the heart. Potato or rice congee can help reduce fire.

Summer is a time of growth and the most active time for metabolism. It is a time of low immunity so it is important to be careful of what you eat and get enough rest.

The second part of summer, which starts around May 21, is called Full Grain. This is a time of much yang qi according to the *Yi Jing/I Ching*. This is a time of much shifting between rain and sun so dampness is a danger so be careful to wear proper clothing. This is a time when rashes happen easily so keep your skin out of the wind to minimize the danger. Some sweating is good because it carries toxins out of the body, but too much sweating makes qi leave the body with the sweat. Minimize air conditioning, especially at night. Avoid icy drinks because they make the inside of the body cold which is bad for the spleen and stomach. Foods that are particularly beneficial in this period are red beans, any type of barley will reduce cold, winter melon, barley soup, any vegetable except eggplant, mung beans in barley soup, mung beans, and tofu. It is okay to eat a little pork, but avoid beef, chicken, and lamb. It is okay to eat fresh water fish, but not salt water fish. Eating mung beans and kelp cooked together into soup is good for hives. Mung beans and barley eaten together benefits the spleen. When preparing seaweed, do not clean it so much that the whiteness comes off. Kelp is excellent for clearing toxins from the body.

Food and Drink

When your body is hot on the outside it is cold on the inside. Therefore, it is very important to not consume cold food or drink in summer. Immunity is lower than rest of year so rest and food is important to eat well particularly during the thirty days after summer equinox. In general, cold food should not be consumed although food directly from the refrigerator is okay since Americans are used to it. A little bit of ice cream is okay. There are many types of food that can make up yin qi, but it is more difficult to make up yang qi. Eating raw red colored foods in the morning or raw onion and red wine in the evening helps circulation. Soaking an onion in red wine for a week then drinking the wine is good for the brain and lessens dementia.

Grains and Beans

Eating only brown rice is best in summer. Eating brown mixed with white is satisfactory, but eating only white is not nutritious enough. Any type of little white beans is good – northern, pinto, etc. Green beans and white bean together is a good combination. Eating mung beans or barley will help release the fire inside and release poisons. When it is hot out eat mung bean soup. To make mung bean soup bring eight units of water to one unit of beans to a boil then simmer until the bean are soft. If you want to sweeten the soup put a few pieces of rock candy in the soup while cooking. Adding brown sugar is acceptable, but it not as good. This is a watery soup which can be eaten hot or cold. Adding couscous to mung bean soup is a good choice. Pearl barley soup is also good if it is cooked a long time. Barley is beneficial for clearing the spleen.

Vegetables

Vegetables such as cucumber, onion, cooked tomato, carrots, and anything with green leaves are an important part of the diet. Sesame seeds on salad is good. Spinach should be cooked because consuming it raw depletes calcium. Cabbage is healthy whether eaten raw or cooked. Garlic is good for preventing bacterial infections like diarrhea. Cucumber that is mixed with raw garlic that has been minced and let to sit for fifteen minutes prevents cancer. Seaweed once a week is good for cleaning your system.

Fruits, Nut, and Seeds

Fresh fruit such as kiwi, grapes, papaya, cherries, blueberries, mixed berries, watermelon, or strawberries with a bit of syrup are highly recommended. If you are sick due to too much internal fire inside then gogi berries are not helpful. Goji is best in fall, winter, and early spring. Using it in summer and long summer can increase fire in your body.

Meat and Fish

Eat only a little meat. Chicken, fish, and duck are best when you do eat meat. Duck is very good for the heart and spleen, especially duck soup which clears the heart.

Other Foods

In terms of spices, a little spicy is fine as is a little bitter such as bitter melon. Salty foods will help the kidneys which tend to be weak at this time of year. Minimal sweet should be eaten in summer. A little honey is good in summer, but molasses should be avoided. Cinnamon in summer is okay, but too much causes fire.

Ginger is very good in summer for most people and a little can be eaten daily, but if your body has lots of yang then ginger can be difficult for your body to handle. Chinese cooking has a lot of ginger and this is very good with meat and seafood. If you are cold, boiling a bit of gingser in water and adding a little brown sugar can be warming.

Beverages

Drinking icy water or other cold drinks should be avoided because they promote dampness in the body which is not good for internal organs. A small amount of beer or wine is okay. You might be hot and sweaty in the summer and a cold drink is appealing, but coldness promotes dampness and prevents the body from releasing toxings. Hot tea makes you sweat and release toxins which is a good thing for the body. Hot water in the morning is beneficial – plain is good, with lemon is better. Cocoa powder with hot water and rather than milk is a good anti-oxidant. Use a bit of sugar, but not honey with the cocoa. It is best to drink this beverage without other foods. How you mix foods and beverages is important because some combinations can create poor chemistry. Cocoa with onions or scallions is one example.

Clothing

No advice specific to summer was given.

Exercise and Qigong

For exercise, practice tai chi outside when the weather is good, especially in the morning when yang qi is strongest. When you practice qigong outside the best location is under yang trees. Humans are a small universe and so are trees. Trees that blossom in yang times are yang and those that blossom in yin times are yin. Evergreen trees are yang as are maple trees. Oak trees are yin. Lots of yang qi will strengthen your spirituality. Sweating is good while doing tai chi because bad energy goes out with the sweat, however, too much sweating is not good. It is best to wait until you cool down after exercise before showering and to use warm, not hot water for your shower. If you sweat a lot during tai ji then sour and bitter foods will help reduce sweating. Doing Five Elements in morning will help clear fire from the heart. In addition, the kidneys and lungs will be stronger because bad energy goes out during the Five Elements heart exercise.

The day of summer solstice is the day when yang ends and yin begins is a special day with lots of movement of energy so it is a particularly good day to do qigong. The best times are at times of change – dawn, dusk, and 11:00-1:00 am and pm. These are the best times on any day including solstice.

Swimming in the ocean is good in summer. The ocean creates negative ions in the water and air. These ions are good energy. Ponds and streams have some negative ions, but not as many as the ocean. Doing qigong near water is good, but not during the heat of the afternoon or when it is windy.

Sleep

Too much sleep in summer is not good for bones. Go to bed late (10:30 or 11:00 pm) and get up early. If you get up early you will receive a lot of yang energy at this time of year. A nap for thirty to sixty minutes is okay. If you take a nap it is best before one o'clock because of flow of yin. Lying down is the best position for napping and lying back in a chair is second best. Leaning forward and resting with your arms on your desk is bad for circulation.

Sexual Activity

The human body is close to the weather, seasons, and atmospheric conditions and when there is a lot of change the chaotic energy conditions are not healthy for the equilibrium of the body. Summer and winter solstice both days to abstain from sex.

Emotions

Just as in spring, avoid anger because it damages your internal energy. Being overly happy can damage the heart.

LONG SUMMER

This is the hottest time of year and is for clearing the spleen. During this season inside of human body has too much fire which is not good for the spleen. Spleen corresponds to earth element and heart corresponds to fire element. If heart is strong, kidney and liver are weak. August usually has very strong good energy; however, sometimes there is a lot of rain which has damp, cold energy which is bad energy. In terms of emotions, be very careful to avoid anger, worry, and stress. Yin is growing and yang is declining. Energy and nutrients are accumulating.

It is important to do qigong daily throughout the year because the environment around you changes daily as does the universe. The hottest three 9-day periods of long summer and the coldest of winter are the best times to improve your body through qigong and tai chi. Why? The extreme heat and cold are challenging and practicing in challenging times is an opportunity for big growth in your practice. The story of Sun Wukong known as the Monkey King, illustrates this truth.

Food and Drink

Eating the proper foods during the time of long summer can release dampness. Do not eat food not directly from refrigerator or have ice cold drinks. Freshly prepared food is the most nutritious food. Food should be eaten within four hours of preparation and leftovers should be avoided during this season.

Grains and Beans

Barley is beneficial for the spleen. Mixing mung beans, rice, couscous together in summer heat helps release bad energy. Oatmeal is good to eat for breakfast especially with peas, raisins, olive oil or green olives. An example of a good dinner soup is couscous with vegetables and adding mung beans that have been brought to a boil then simmered until they break open is an option. Oatmeal with peas and carrots and a bit of olive oil and raisins is good. Try it with pickles or green olives. Couscous soup made with one part couscous to three or four parts water and cooked for thirty to forty minutes then covered and cooled is a healthy dinner soup. A little rock sugar can be added if you wish. Mung beans soup made by bringing them to a boil then simmering for an hour or two until they break open is also a good summer soup. Mung beans, rice, and couscous helps heat to go out of your body.

Vegetables

Vegetables such as shallots, onions, or green beans are helpful. Eggplant is good for blood and helps control cholesterol. Cutting fresh garlic, letting it sit fifteen minutes then put it raw into salad or other food is helpful. Salad should be eaten within four hours of preparation if it has dressing on it. Leftover rice undergoes changes inside that make it hard for internal organs to use and is never good to eat. In this season leftovers of any kind are not good. Cooking garlic removes the nutrition. Seaweed once every two weeks clears the body.

Fruits, Nut, and Seeds

Examples of fruits particularly useful during summer heat are kiwi, cherry, grapes, and papaya. Blueberries are especially helpful for your eyes. Watermelons that are refrigerated lose half of their nutritional value. Watermelon is very yin so it is good for reducing fire, but this value is lost if the watermelon is refrigerated. The white part of watermelon rind boiled with a small amount of salt can help rind heal cough. This is also good for kidney.

Meat and Fish

Restrict the amount of meat consumed.

Other Foods

A little sugar is okay in this season. Spices make fire and are not good for the young.

Beverages

Drink water before eating.

Clothing

In mid-August long summer begins to change to fall and the weather begins to cool. This is a time to gradually add clothes.

Exercise and Qigong

Doing both qigong and tai chi daily is best, but if you do not have time for both prioritize qigong. Do not do tai chi if you sweat too much because original qi/yuan qi can be depleted. Start tai chi, but stop if you sweat too much in order to avoid depletion. Five elements qigong is to clear the heart. When you practice qigong at home during "too hot" season make sure a fan is not blowing hard, no air conditioning if that is possible because during qigong you are especially sensitive to cold because your cells are open. Strong flow of wind such as being between an open door and an open window is to be avoided.

Qigong sweating is different from regular sweating. It helps toxins leave your body. If you sweat during qigong in long summer your body will be healthier in winter because of the toxins that were released. Wait a while before showering after qigong to give your cells time to close. A lot of exercise during long summer is not desirable.

Sleep

The optimum sleep pattern is to wake up early and go to bed late. When the switch from long summer to fall begins in mid-August, continue to wake up early and begin going to bed earlier. Do not sleep with a fan blowing directly at you. Avoid sleeping outside during this time because the dampness can be drawn into your body.

Sexual Activity

No advice specific to long summer was given.

Emotions

The heart needs calmness particularly in long summer. It is particularly important to have positive emotions in long summer. Your mood influences hormones so being happy contributes to the release of desirable hormones. A few years ago there was an experiment in which a Japanese man spoke lovingly to water. He used his intention to create crystals. He also talked negatively to water. The water receiving loving talk formed beautiful crystals while unattractive crystals were formed by water that was exposed to negative talk. This is important for humans since a baby is 85% water, adults 70%, and seniors 65%. These suggests that it is important to speak kindly to others and to keep your emotions clear.

FALL SEASON

Fall is the season when nature is turning from hot to cold and the time when light and darkness equalize. Yin builds and yang fades as daylight shortens. This is a time to conserve qi and gather yin and yang so life needs to slow down and close a bit as we move toward winter which is the time to store. Since yang decreases in fall it is important to conserve yang energy especially if you are older because yang begins to decrease after the age of forty so it must be conserved. Engage in physical activity, but do not overdo it. Focus on developing spirit. If you feel tired by activity, then decrease activity. The key is listening to your body. If you're middle aged fall is a good time of year to cut back activity to maintain your yang qi. A lot of travel drains yang because of the schedule changes. Retired people travel in fall, but it is really not a good idea because changing your schedule is draining. Spring and summer are good times to be active.

The increasing dryness of fall makes it a good time for clearing lung. Lungs are associated with metal. When you are stressed or worried it impacts your lungs. Therefore, control your emotions. If you cough a lot or you believe your lungs are not strong face west when doing qigong. If your lungs are good it helps kidney, therefore, clearing lungs now will make kidneys strong in the winter. If your feet have pain your kidneys might be weak.

Overall, fall is the season to strengthen stomach. Stomach energy is very important for health and long life. Fall is a season of contraction which makes it easier for stomach illness to occur. If you eat a little and are not hungry it means you do not have enough stomach energy which is not good. Caring for the spleen in first ten days of fall is important because yin is building and spleen transforms energy for blood and bodily fluids which are yin in nature.

Fall is not the time of kidney yet it is important to begin clearing the kidney now so it will be prepared for storage of yang qi in winter. Everyone has yin and yang. They are not just substances. Yang has yin, yin has yang. There is much change and sometimes there is too much of one and lack of the other. There are times of balance, however, it is normal for the balance to change quickly. Problems in other organs can be felt in early stages, but if you can feel a kidney problem it has progressed beyond the beginning stage. A sign of kidney needing care is tiredness at the end of the day. Jing of kidney is original qi received from parents. The amount of qi obtained from parents determines the length of life. There are two types of qi deficiency – yang qi, yin qi. Cold hands especially palm lo gong are symptomatic of yang deficiency while sweating when it is cold is symptomatic of yin qi deficiency. There are few foods that make up deficiency of yang qi. Lamb, Chinese ginseng, and deer antler in tea are among the few foods that can make up yang qi. Many foods can make up a deficiency of yin qi – for example black beans, dates, black sesame, mulberry.

The second period of fall, chū shǔ, is a short period of heat before temperatures begin to cool. It is the time of most danger from coldness. Air conditioning, icy drinks, ice cream, and cold-natured foods such as watermelon can be eaten in limited quantities for most people. People with stomach problems should eat none.

The fifth period of fall, hán lù, is when enough coldness in the environment has developed so that wearing two pair of pants is good. It is still fall and time for caring for lungs yet close enough to winter that you must care for kidneys by keeping warm. This is especially important as an individual becomes older.

Food and Drink

Too much food makes it difficult for spleen to do its work so an overall guideline is to eat to 70% full. Start each day with a nutritious breakfast. Having honey in morning or sesame seeds and almonds for breakfast will help avoid constipation. At lunchtime eat to 100% full so you will have enough energy for the afternoon. For dinner eat to 70-80% full. Soup at dinnertime is recommended. Avoid cold beverages and cold food throughout this season because they can damage the spleen and stomach. If you care for those organs your lungs will be stronger. White is the color for this season and white foods are good including foods that are white underneath a skin of a different color.

Grains and Beans

A variety of beans – red, black, and white - is good in fall. Simmering black and white beans for two to three hours into a soup then adding vegetables and dried mushrooms that have been soaked. Mung beans should not be eaten in the fall. Millet for dinner is good for the whole body. Chinese eat it alone, but Americans like it with meat or in soup. Adding a little brown sugar or a chopped up hard-boiled egg to millet is ok. White beans and sticky rice is a healthy fall combination. Eat a little brown rice, but not white. Millet soup for dinner can help in this season if you have trouble sleeping. Barley is the best grain. Barley and white beans is a good combination to benefit spleen and to make up qi. White beans make up for lack of qi while red or black beans make up lack in blood.

Vegetables

Vegetables particularly good for fall are eggplant, green beans, tomato, cauliflower, and carrots. Daikon radish is especially helpful if simmered with nori for an hour as a soup. Fresh, raw garlic prevents cancer. Slice it and expose to air for fifteen minutes before eating. Onion, especially fresh, is healthy for joints. Winter melon is a vegetable available in Asian groceries.

Fruits, Nuts, and Seeds

Gogi berries (also called wolf berries) clear the kidneys. Six or seven water chestnuts in soup is good for kidneys. Although it is best not to eat a lot of fruit in fall, especially fruits that are cold in nature several fruits are helpful in fall when eaten in moderation. Pears and persimmons are good for the lungs and for reducing mucus as well as for tendons and joints. If you have cough, boil pears for twenty minutes with a bit of honey. Raspberry and blueberries help wake up yin energy. Peaches, apples, pineapple, and oranges are helpful, but not tangerines. Banana and watermelon both have a cold nature so they should be eaten in limited amounts in the fall. Apples with cinnamon is warming and is beneficial in fall.

Meat and Fish

Some people feel cold in this season. Eating a little bit of meat can help by creating internal warmth. Beef, chicken, or fish are the best choices. Beginning late in the fall, eating lamb is good for improving immunity and for blood. Lamb in soup is the best way to eat lamb this time of year. Eating meat at lunch rather than dinner is preferable.

Other Foods

Only a little spicy food should be eaten in fall because too much damages the bodily fluids (*jīn yè*). Minimize the amount of ginger you consume because too much can cause qi to leak out of your body. Lung likes some sweet so sweets are good in fall, but too much is not good for liver. A little sour, not too much tart is fine as is a little spice. Bitter is not helpful in this season. The lung likes spicy, but too much can damage it. Metal supports water and controls wood, but too much spice makes it hard for metal to carry out these functions. Ginger is okay in fall if you are sick. Sour helps the spleen and spleen helps the lung.

Beverages

What you drink in the fall is very important because the danger in this season is that the increasingly dry energy from the earth, which is yin in nature, can easily consume bodily fluids (*jīn yè*) can be consumed easily. For example, it is easy to become constipated in fall. Some people develop a cough due to lungs becoming too dry. Blood pressure problems can develop from internal dryness... Drinking about a half cup of warm or room temperature water when you first get up helps clear poisons from your internal organs. Eat breakfast later. During the day drinking tea is best, however, drinking water is good as long as the water is not cold and has no ice. Adding lemon to water is very good. If cholesterol is not high, a small cup of cocoa powder in hot water with a little sugar is okay to drink each day. The cocoa is an antioxidant. Drink a total of eight cups of water a day. It is best to drink the eight cups on a schedule of four or five times rather than whenever you feel like drinking. It is best to drink thirty to sixty minutes before lunch or dinner. Drinking water with or immediately after a meal can be unhelpful because it dilutes digestive acids.

Clothing

The key principle for this fall is to keep the inside of your body warm - especially lungs. Do not rush to put on more clothes as the weather cools. Take care to keep yourself warm in the morning and evening. Always keep your feet warm. Wear socks. As it gets cooler, wear more clothes evening and morning. Dress in layers so you can shift from warmer clothes in the morning to fewer clothes in the warmer afternoon and warmer clothes as the evening cools. Examples are wearing a tank top under a shirt or wearing a vest. Do not be concerned about covering your arms as long as your torso is covered. It is easy for the waist to get cold so be sure to keep it warm.

Exercise & Qigong

For exercise enjoy nature such as going hiking. While exercise is important, it is important not to have too much activity because yin is building, yang is diminishing. The weather is good. The best time to practice tai chi is upon waking. Any time before noon is good since this is the time of day when there is most yang.

Building yang qi in fall is good so that there will be enough to store for the winter. Yang qi can be built through standing qigong. It can also be built during le xin gong by thinking of light going to the mingmen or warming it by imaging light melting snow on a mountain. You won't feel it, but the mingmen is receiving qi. There is a relationship between the mingmen and kidney so helping the mingmen helps the kidney.

Sleep

Early to sleep and early to wake is the optimal sleep pattern because once qi rises to far it is too late to control it. Early morning has good yin so it is particularly good time to get up, but if you sleep too late you miss this potential benefit. Getting up late in the fall contributes to coughing and mucous production. Going to bed late consumes yang energy and this is not good for kidney.

Sexual Activity

Decrease sexual activity as yin decreases because. Too much sex drains kidneys.

Emotions

Sadness can damage lungs. Worry can damage kidneys. Sometimes a western diagnosis can cause fear or worry, but for optimal health you need emotional peace. Western physicians look for problems in organs and may test a kidney for infection or cancer. Chinese physicians are interested in kidney having enough jing, qi, and shen and enough yin qi and yang qi. Having these in balance will prevent problems. Caring for the kidney by avoiding fear and worry is part of preventing problems since both deplete kidney.

Other

Soaking your feet in water that is hot to the touch (no hotter than 113^0F) will help circulation. Do not add Epsom salts because the water opens pores and bad might go in. Water should be up to knees if possible because there is an acupressure point below knee on outside of knee. Massage your feet while they're in the water for about twenty minutes. Doing this immediately before bedtime is best.

WINTER SEASON

Yin and yang must be balanced in all seasons. In fall and winter there is an increasing amount of yin. During winter yin and yang become separated from each other since yin rests in the earth and yang ascends to heaven. This split makes life very hard for all living things. Nature and all living things close and store. Snakes and other animals hibernate and trees lose their leaves and rest. Snake symbolizes yin. Yin snake has no movement in winter and people are the same. The human spirit needs to rest in the winter. Clear your spirit by staying calm and relaxed.

Winter is divided into six parts – Winter Begins, Small Snow, Big Snow, Winter Solstice, Small Cold, Big Cold. Winter has nine periods of nine days each. Each of the first three periods grow increasingly cold. Warming in nature begins during the fifth set of nine days. Birds begin returning and worms resume their activity. The winter solstice is the first day of a twelve day period in which it is particularly important to accumulate good qi and to clear the kidney. At this time of year the universe has only a small amount of yang and so does your body. On the day of the solstice yang begins to build in the universe as well as in your body. Yang is stored in the kidney. It can be thought of as yang beginning to grow in the way and newborn baby grows.

Winter is the best time among seasons to take care of health. It is a good time to clear the kidney. Winter is the time to close and store. Winter is a time to support the increase and clear yin in your body. Clearing yin makes it easier to store yang. Winter is the time of kidneys which have a water nature. Kidneys store your essences, jing and qi, so caring for them is very important. The kidney and *mingmen* is important because it is where development of the fetus begins.

When thinking about how to care for your kidneys you should consider how to accumulate yang qi, avoid depleting jing and qi, and making up any existing lack. Yang qi can be accumulated through the food you eat and qigong. It can be depleted by too much exercise, too much sexual activity, and emotional upset. During the twelve days immediately following the winter solstice it is advisable to abstain from sexual activity. Making up for any lack during this time can help your body be strong all year. If you sweat a lot even with little or no exercise it could be from a lack of qi. The twelve days after solstice are particularly good for filling this lack. Women must be particularly careful of their blood and men of their jing. Jing is consumed when semen is used. *Jing qi* and *yuan qi* are being stored in the kidney this season so it is particularly important to keep them warm. Coldness depletes your *yuan qi*.

Of the six evil influences, cold is the most influential in the winter.

In winter it is cold outside yet warm inside the body. Internal cold can damage kidney qi or make it leave the body so you must keep your body warm to prevent cold from entering the body. Physical problems that are most likely to occur in winter are stroke, high blood pressure, or paint in the legs were stomach. The most common reason for these problems is failure to stay warm. The three most important things to keep warm are the *bai hui* on the crown your head, your neck and chest, and your feet. Wear a hat to keep your *baihui* and head warm so wear a hat. If you do not wear a hat it is easier to have a stroke or heart problem because the cold interrupts the circulation. Thirty percent of your body heat can be lost through your head. If the weather is a very cold, it is possible to lose even more heat from your body. Wear a scarf to keep your and chest warm. If the chest becomes cold it can trigger heart problems. Keeping your feet warm in this season is particularly important to prevent injury to your kidneys and *mingmen*. Your feet are far from your heart so it is easy for them to become cold. Soaking your feet in hot water before going to bed is particularly beneficial for keeping your feet and body warm. Some people should soak their feet in hot water every day. Water up to the knee is best because there is an important meridian just below the knee. There is a close connection between back pain and the kidney meridian in the foot therefore, keeping the feet warm helps relieve back pain. Feet connect to gall bladder and liver as well as many minor meridians.

If your kidneys are weak in the winter, then you might have liver problems in the spring. If you become tired in the afternoon it could be a symptom of weakness in the kidney. If your body is sick or weak winter is a good time to eat foods that will restore your body. Your body can be restored through the food you eat the beverages you drink and getting the proper amounts of sleep.

If you take care of yourself now, you will be stronger in the spring. In each season opposite conditions exist in the body from what exists in nature. Kidneys can be strengthened in winter through daily qigong, increasing the amount of qigong, daily five elements exercise, and daily taiji. Although amount of exercise is decreased in the winter you cannot do too much qigong or taiji. Daily practice will clear your body and balance yin and yang. Eat black colored food to make up yin such as black wood ear fungus which lowers cholesterol, black beans, pecans, walnuts, peanuts, black sesame seeds, blackberries, and mulberries.

Food and Drink

Each person's body is different so each has different   food needs, however, there are some general principles that guide what to eat. Eat all types of food in balance in the winter. If your hands are cold it can be from too much yin qi. This happens more frequently for women. Foods can be used to kill warmth and increase yang.

Anything except canned food is okay in the winter. if your stomach is okay, but you must be more selective if your stomach is weak. Winter is the time to supplement yang through the food you eat and to clear your kidneys. Ginseng can be useful for making up a lack of qi. American ginseng is weaker than the ginseng grown in China or Korea. American ginseng is good for the heart. Chinese and Korean ginseng is good for the stomach, spleen, lung, and kidney. If your nose bleeds easily it could be from not enough qi. Up to three grams of American ginseng might help. Use the powdered form in qi or cook the root into rice, congee, or chicken soup. Soup is good to eat in the evening. Start the soup with water then add what you want. Soup warms stomach and cuts down portions you eat.

Grains and Beans

Sticky or sweet rice is very good for warming the inside of the body during this time of coldness. Red and black beans are the best beans for this time of year.

Vegetables

Eat plenty of vegetables especially carrots. Eat any kind of mushrooms as long as you cook them. Parsley can prevent colds, onions, garlic, chili peppers. Lotus root in soup.

Fruits, Nuts, and Seeds

Walnuts are helpful as are up to ten chestnuts in rice soup or chicken soup. Gogi berries, which are also called wolf berries, are good for clearing kidneys. Dried dragon eyes which are a Chinese fruit, Blackberries, mulberries, black sesame seeds, chestnuts,

Meat and Fish

Some meat is okay. Fish and shrimp are the best choices. Shrimp helps make up yang, however, it should never be eaten with foods that are high in vitamin C such as tomato or citrus fruits. Shrimp is particularly good with leeks because they bring out the best in each other. You can stir fry them together or use them as stuffing for dumplings. Chicken, turkey, and duck are okay. Beef and pork should be limited. Duck has a lot of fat, but it is not a bad fat. Lamb is the best meat to eat this time of year. A soup of lamb with carrots and daikon radish is particularly good. Do not drink tea or use vinegar on a day that you eat lamb because that makes an unhealthy chemical combination. If you cough a lot soup made with chicken or duck can be helpful.

Other Foods

Eggs can be eaten only three times a week by senior people, but daily by young people. Avoid eating too much salt. Although the kidney likes salt it depletes your yuan qi.

Beverages

Green tea should be drunk daily to clear the body. Milk can be consumed daily only in this season. Some people use herb drinks that provide energy, but this can provide too much yang and creates imbalance so you must be careful of what you drink. It is best to not drink fluids in the evening since it increases the need to urinate during the night which makes the kidneys work too hard.

Clothing

Wear two layers of pants in the winter. Keeping your feet warm protects your kidneys. Do not wear shoes with open heels in winter. Wear thick your soles on your shoes.

Exercise and Qigong

Exercise in moderation in winter avoid depleting qi and other internal energies and to conserve yang during this increasingly yin time of the year, but some exercise is good. Each person can make her or his own choice of type of activity. Exercising in fresh air is best. Tai chi is helpful in the winter but you should stop if you become too sweaty because too much sweating can deplete the body.

Do *le xin gong* or *xiao zhou tian* qigong daily as well as *gù shèn bŭ xŭ gong* which is a special qigong to clear the kidneys. If you do qigong at night soak your feet in hot water first, but leave time in between the two activities. Soaking the whole body in a hot tub is acceptable rather than soaking just the feet.

Sleep

Go to bed early and rise after the sun rises helps in the care of your yang qi especially if you're older. Early sleep protects and accumulates yang qi. Waking up late clears your yin qi. The warmth of bed contributes to the processes that support qi. Sleeping in the nude is good at any time of the year because it allows better circulation and allows the skin to breathe. This is particularly helpful in the winter. Be sure to cover yourself with enough warm blankets to keep yourself warm. If you do decide to sleep wearing clothes they should be made of cotton or other natural fibers. Sleeping on your side with your legs and all arms beds is best. Sleeping on your right side is better for your heart, but it is okay to sleep on either side. In winter keeps the window closed at night because it will be too cold when you get up to use the bathroom. The temperature of the room at night should be 68-70^0 for younger people and70^0 four senior people. If the temperature of the room is colder than these ideal temperatures put clothes on if you get up to use the bathroom. If you wake up early, don't open the windows until 9:00 am. If you have a hard time sleeping, do qigong in the morning rather than at night

Sexual Activity

Too much sex depletes the *yuanqi* in your kidney so it is best to abstain or be moderate to protect the kidney qi/*yuanqi*. Young and middle aged people can have a moderate amount of sex. For older people less sexual activity is advisable in winter in order to preserve yang energy. The key is to avoid depleting your body through too much sexual activity. Too much sex means opening the body in ways it closes for winter. Making semen and using energy for sexual activity depletes energy more during this season than other season. This applies to men and women, but men are depleted more since they make semen.

Emotions

Fear is the main emotion related to kidneys. Worry can damage your kidneys and this can damage the body. If a western physician tells you you are sick do not worry even if the illness is serious. Fear can weaken the kidneys. If your kidneys are weak fear can increase. Therefore, take care of your kidneys to minimize problems caused by fear.

Other

There is a relationship between the ears and kidneys. A lot of loud sound tires the ears and is not good for kidneys.

ABOUT THE AUTHOR

Janice has been practicing tai chi and qigong since 1998. She was a student at Center for Harmony for eight years. Over time, her taking class notes for her personal use morphed into documenting class lectures for Shifu. Janice is the author of *Healing Bodies, Healing Hearts with Tai Chi Chuan and Qigong*. She was the ghost writer for Lijun Cheng's "My Lotus Grown Out of Mud" published in *The Power of Grieving – A Stronger You* by Maryjane Boggins-Atkins.

Cover photography is by Margery Gerard.

Made in the USA
Middletown, DE
12 January 2018